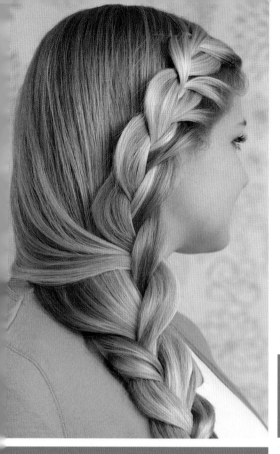
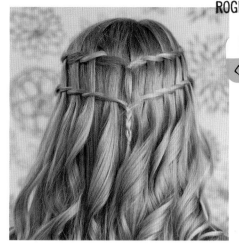
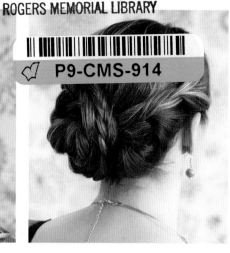
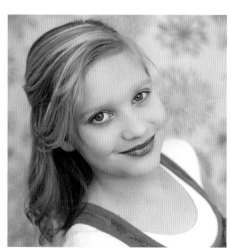
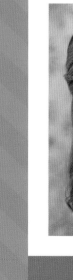
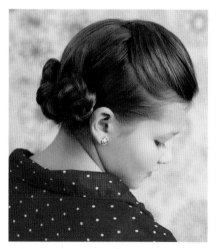

AMAZING HAIRSTYLES

from EASY to ELEGANT

STEP-BY-STEP **STYLES** FOR ANY AGE OR OCCASION

BECKY PORTER

PHOTOGRAPHY BY KATIE ROBERTS

PLAIN SIGHT PUBLISHING | AN IMPRINT OF CEDAR FORT, INC. | SPRINGVILLE, UTAH

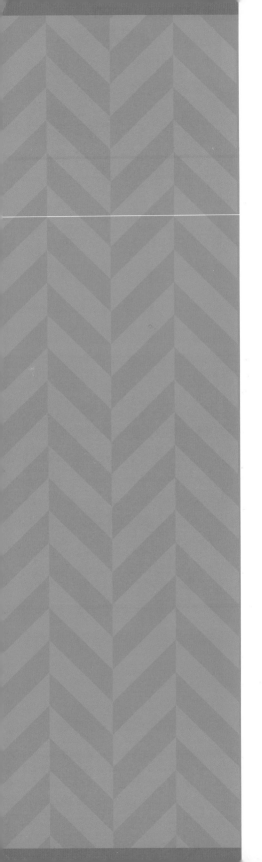

ISBN 13: 978-1-4621-1503-7

Published by Plain Sight Publishing,
an imprint of Cedar Fort, Inc.
2373 W. 700 S., Springville, UT 84663
Distributed by Cedar Fort, Inc., www.cedarfort.com

LIBRARY OF CONGRESS CATALOGING-IN-PUBLICATION DATA

Porter, Rebecca, 1976- author.
Amazing hairstyles from easy to elegant / Rebecca Porter ;
photography by Katie Roberts.
    pages cm
Includes bibliographical references and index.
ISBN 978-1-4621-1503-7 (alk. paper)
1. Hairdressing. 2. Hairstyles. I. Roberts, Katie, 1975- illustrator. II. Title.

TT972.P59 2014
646.7'24--dc23
                                        2014022512

Cover and page design by Angela D. Baxter and Lacey Hathaway
Cover design © 2014 by Lyle Mortimer
Edited by Eileen Leavitt

Photography by Katie Roberts
www.lampshadestudio.com

Printed in the United States of America

10   9   8   7   6   5   4   3   2   1

Printed on acid-free paper

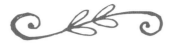

"AS ONE WHO GREW UP with a mom who was a "master hair braider," I just assumed that it would be easy for me to do my own girls' hair. Once they had hair long enough for me to play with, I realized that I really had no idea what I was doing, and my girls usually had their hair in a ponytail. Thankfully, *Amazing Hairstyles* came to my rescue! Becky's crystal-clear directions and beautiful step-by-step pictures walk you through each hairstyle, making it easy to follow along and re-create for yourself. There are so many fun styles that I was inspired to attempt and this book makes it possible for me to do. I would highly recommend this book to anyone who has ever wanted to learn how to do hair and wasn't sure where to start or just needs some fresh ideas of new hairstyles. This book is absolutely amazing."

CAMILLE BECKSTRAND,
from *Six Sisters' Stuff*, WWW.SIXSISTERSTUFF.COM

"I HAVE BEEN A BIG FAN of *Babes in Hairland* for a long time. As a mother of two girls, who loved to get all dolled up, I have found the blog to be a lifesaver. Her easy-to-understand tutorials have taken me from barely knowing how to braid to creating hair masterpieces! I am always so amazed at the fun, innovative, and beautiful hairstyles that Becky comes up with and I'm thrilled that I can finally have her tutorials in book form. Whether you're starting from square one or are an experienced hairstylist, you're sure to find many creative hairstyles for any occasion."

MARIEL WANGSGARD,
from *Or So She Says*, WWW.ORSOSHESAYS.COM

"BECKY PORTER is one of the most talented and creative 'styling' moms we've had the pleasure of working with since we first launched Curlformers nearly eight years ago. She initially bought them to curl her daughters' hair and wanted to experiment with a more gentle, 'heat-free' option. Over the years, Becky has used the different sized-Curlformers to create an array of stunning styles on her lovely girls as well as herself and her friends, which she has written about and videoed for her *Babes in Hairland* blog, providing inspiration for women and little princesses around the world. To write a book bursting with easy-to-follow tutorials, tips and techniques to create styles that are easy, fast, elegant, or complex—the choice is endless—is a natural progression for this hair-obsessed, fun-loving mom."

WWW.CURLFORMERS.COM

"I'M LOOKING FORWARD to the release of *Amazing Hairstyles* by Becky Porter. Becky is a very talented hairstylist who has made her mark in the blogging world and is rightfully is taking her place in the bound world in the form of *Amazing Hairstyles* the book. This beautiful collection of styles is going to be a much-needed tool in the house of every mother, teen, and child. What a great way to have in hand a collection of styles to choose from for daily hairstyles and even for a more elegant occasion. It will be a cherished addition to any girl's favorite books."

JENN NELSON,
from *Girly Do Hairstyles*, WWW.GIRLYDOHAIRSTYLES.COM

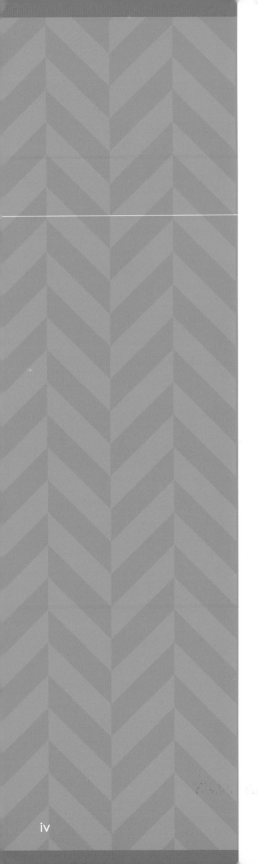

CONTENTS

CONTENTS

ACKNOWLEDGMENTS

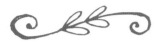

THANK YOU to a kind and loving Heavenly Father for daily miracles, big and small.

To my three sweet and amazing girls—"Goose," "Bug," and "Bee." Without you, none of this would have been possible. Ee-Lee-Voo

To Mike, my PC #1 for always believing in me. For putting up with all the estrogen in the house and allowing our bedroom and bathroom to be overrun by hair stuff. Thank you for being my best friend as well as biggest cheerleader and support through this whole adventure.

Thanks Katie Horst Pead Roberts for still being the fun and crazy girl I met in Deutschland all those years ago. Thank you for reminding me everything would be OK—then and now. Thank you for sharing your amazing photography skills with me and the rest of the world.

A huge thank you to all my beautiful models: Adelaide, Alayna, Aliyah, Brooklyn, Hailey, Jamie, Jill, Liberty, Lindsay, McKayla, Melody, Neva, Raquelle, Remington, Shay, and Stephanie. Thank you for your patience and willingness to help make my dream a reality. And thank you to their moms for lending me their cute daughters!

Also, thank you Haley Miller Swan for finding my blog and to all the talented staff at Cedar Fort for making my dream of writing a book come true.

And of course, to my wonderful blog readers—thank you for returning time and time again.

INTRODUCTION

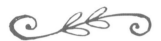

HI THERE AND WELCOME! If you've picked up this book, I will assume it's because you are interested in learning how to do hair, either on yourself or others, are looking for inspiration, or just love looking at great hairstyles.

This book is unique, because regardless of if you are a hair novice or an expert, there is something here for everyone. Whether you are a school-aged girl hoping to find something your mom can do in the morning before school, a tween starting to experiment with your hair, a teen who is heading to prom, or a mom hoping to learn how to do her own hair or more than just pigtails and braids in your daughter's hair—you've come to the right place!

I am the mother to three wonderful daughters. Having three girls means I do a lot of hair each day. I started blogging and sharing hairstyles I created when they were little girls, because at the time, there was little to no help available online, and books at the library were extremely outdated or didn't teach me anything new. I figured if I was out looking for hair ideas to do in my daughter's hair, other moms must be as well. But, in the end, the real reason I do their hair and have created so many hairstyles over the years is because of the one-on-one quality time it allows me to have

with them. In today's busy world and crazy schedules we all keep, I cherish the time I spend doing my girls' hair each day. And though they probably won't admit it, they like the time too, because they know they've got my full attention. If you're just getting into doing your daughter's hair, I highly encourage it! Time with our children is fleeting so I would invite you to spend a few extra minutes in the morning to do a little something more than a ponytail!

You should also probably know that I have no "formal" training in the world of cosmetology or anything of that nature. And quite frankly, until about seven years ago I had no idea how to even French braid. I am not a hairdresser—I'm just someone who is passionate about creating hairstyles and sharing them with others. That being said, if I can go from not being able to do more than pigtails and braids on my girls to sharing these amazing styles in a book with you, then anyone can learn how to do hair. Learning how to do hair is a skill that can be learned by anyone. You just have to practice and have patience with yourself.

So what are you waiting for? Grab a comb and someone who will let you play with their hair and let's go create some amazing hairstyles together!

CHAPTER 1

Tips, Essential Supplies & More

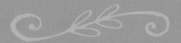

*Styling tools and supplies we used to achieve the hairstyles
throughout the book and my two cents about them.*

MESSAGE TO MOMS & CAREGIVERS

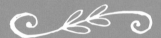

WHEN I FIRST started blogging and my girls were younger, I was often asked how I got my girls to hold still while I combed their hair. The answer is "I didn't." I just learned to work fast on a moving target! I did, however, do things to distract them. I always had them up on my bathroom counter, and just being in front of the mirror was a big help. I gave them different combs or hair things to play with. They also liked to play with our spray bottle of water.

The biggest suggestion I would offer to moms or caregivers of little girls is to start doing their hair as young as you can so it becomes part of the routine. By so doing, you will usually be met with less resistance as they get older. When they are babies, even if they just have just a little bit of hair, it's never too young to start. Put a stretchy little headband on them or if they have enough hair, make a little tiny "spout" of a ponytail on top. When my youngest was a baby I would lay her on her diaper table, put a little gel in her hair and brush it into a tiny little curl on top and add a cute stretchy headband.

As they become more mobile, you can also put them in their high chair and give them a few snacks or toys to play with while you do their hair. I know moms who have certain toys designated just for "hair time." I know of other moms who turn on a TV show or let their daughter play with their cell phone or tablet to distract during hair time. Experiment and try different things until you find what works best for you and your child. With the small amount of hair they may have, doing little pigtails or ponies that connect with elastics to keep baby hair out of the eyes is a good starting point.

As they get older it's fun to play little games, sing songs, practice counting and saying the ABC's and even just talk with them while you do their hair. It truly can be cherished one-on-one time. I have had so many moms tell me that their time together doing hair has improved their relationship, and by creating cute and fun styles it has also helped boost their self-image. It's a win-win! They really do grow up too fast! Remember—in the end, it's about the time you spend with your child that matters the most—not so much the hair!

HAIR TERMS

THESE ARE A FEW hair terms I use throughout the book. They may or may not be official, but this way you know what I am talking about.

When describing where to position something in a hairstyle, or where to start a part, these are three areas that I use a lot.

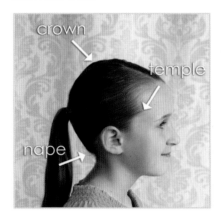

BOUFFANT OR POOF

An area on the crown or top of the head that has been backcombed to create volume. It also helps give the appearance of fuller thicker hair.

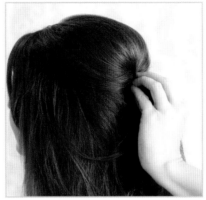

FLY-AWAYS

This may be a term only I use, but these are also known as wispy loose hairs that stick out of a style. These can be caused by baby hairs, split ends, uneven lengths, etc. If you want a style to look clean and neat, fly-aways are not our friends. Help tame them by misting hair with water or use some kind of product or hair spray while styling. However, if you are trying to achieve a messy and carefree style, they only add to it!

ROTATION

This is the term I use when you have completed one "round" or revolution of a braid. For example, in a regular 3-strand braid you always cross the right strand over the middle strand, and then the left strand over the middle strand. That is what I consider one *rotation*. You repeat this over and over to create a braid.

TAIL

The ends of a braid or section of hair with which you might be working.

TEASE OR BACKCOMB

To comb a section of hair repeatedly towards the scalp, causing the hair to tangle and knot up, is what's referred to as backcombing. It is often done on top of the head or crown. This is done to create volume in a hairstyle. It's a great trick if you are working with thin or fine hair.

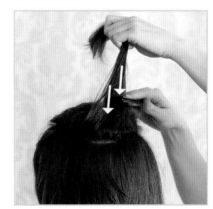

STYLING TOOLS

IF YOUR INITIAL THOUGHT when looking through this book is, "I can't do these hairstyles, I don't have expensive tools like my stylist," or, "I just can't do hair—period," then let me remind you: I'm not a cosmetologist/stylist and have no formal training, but I have learned to do hair. Second, I am proof that when doing hair, you don't necessarily need the most expensive or top-of-the-line tools to get the job done. Nor do you have to be a cosmetologist to create amazing hairstyles.

Let me share a little story with you. About a year ago, because I love updos and fancy hair, I had the opportunity to attend a hair class focusing on bridal and wedding hairstyles. It was taught by an amazingly talented professional stylist, and all others in attendance were licensed cosmetologists. Then there was me—the cute little "hair blogger!" All the cosmetologists arrived with suitcases on wheels full of their fancy and expensive salon equipment. All I had with me was a bag with my few basic combs, my old and ugly flat iron and curling iron I'd bought from Wal-Mart,

some pomade, and a bottle of Suave hair spray. I started to feel like I'd made a huge mistake coming to the class. That was, until the stylist proceeded to share the things she used to create her amazing styles that appear in magazines and all over the internet. None of the tools or hair techniques she used were much fancier than what I was using and she proceeded to create gorgeous hairstyles with them for the class. That's when I realized I wasn't crazy thinking I could create beautiful styles with my basic tools and I definitely shouldn't feel intimidated! Now obviously, she has skills that have been learned from years of doing hair on a daily basis, but the point is, she didn't have the most expensive styling tools or product and still created incredible styles.

You too can create amazing hairstyles with tools that don't cost an arm and leg. Following are the basic hair tools that were used to create the styles for this book as well as most of the styles on my blog. However, you don't need all of them for every style. Just double check you have everything you need before starting a hairstyle!

SPRAY BOTTLE OF WATER

HAIR PINS

BOBBY PINS
DIFFERENT SIZES AND COLORS

CLAW CLIPS
MULTIPLE SIZES

HAIR ELASTICS & PONYTAIL HOLDERS

WIDE-TOOTH COMB

BASIC COMB

RAT-TAIL COMB

BACK-COMBING COMB

TOPSY TAIL

CURLING IRON

STRAIGHTENER/ FLAT IRON

CURLERS

ACCESSORIES
HEADBANDS, CLIPS, ETC.

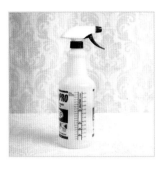

WATER BOTTLE

This is a must have—especially when working on younger girls' hair. If you want to avoid fly-aways and make hair look smooth and neat, a good water bottle is priceless. If you want a good water bottle, buy one from your hardware store. You want one that is technically meant for mixing water with some sort of cleaning solution and most likely has measurements up the side of it. I know from experience that if you buy one of those little ones from the dollar store or elsewhere, it won't last long and it won't work very well at all. The one pictured cost me under $2 from the local hardware store. Fill it with water and you are good to go!

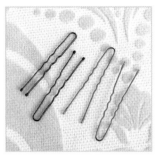

HAIR PINS

These are not the same as bobby pins. They are U-shaped and are used more in updos when you literally want to "pin" hair in place. They don't clamp shut and hold hair like bobby pins do. They come in a few colors to match hair color. They are also great to use when making your own accessories for an updo. It's so easy to hot glue pearls or other jewels to them and place them throughout your hairstyle. I recommend buying these from a beauty supply store because they tend to be sturdier.

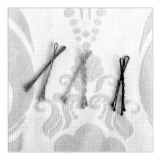

BOBBY PINS
(ALSO KNOWN AS A HAIR GRIP OR KIRBY)

Contrary to what you may believe, all bobby pins are not created equal. If you find yourself using tons of bobby pins to hold your hair in place—chances are it's because you are using cheap bobby pins. I know I talked about not having to spend a lot of money on hair tools, but if you want your hair to hold when using bobby pins—don't just buy ones that come on a card of 50 from the dollar store. Spend an extra few dollars and buy ones from a beauty supply store. Invest in some today. You will thank me later!

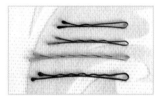

You probably knew that bobby pins come in different colors, but did you know they also come in different sizes? Small bobby pins are wonderful for working with toddler hair, fine hair, or when needing to secure a small amount of hair in a style.

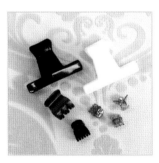

CLAW CLIPS

Rarely do I use a claw clip as an accessory in a hair style. Instead, they are great for holding hair out of the way or temporarily securing hair while a hairstyle is in process. They are especially helpful when working with toddler hair or small sections of hair. I use them to keep braids and twists from unraveling when I need to work on a different section of hair.

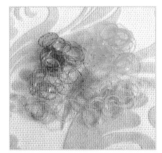

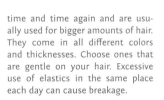

HAIR ELASTICS & PONYTAIL HOLDERS

You may refer to these differently, but most everyone needs them at some point to secure their hair. Small elastics are usually used for securing small sections of hair and are good for one use only. The ones I use are about as big around as a nickel or dime. Whereas, covered ponytail holders can be used time and time again and are usually used for bigger amounts of hair. They come in all different colors and thicknesses. Choose ones that are gentle on your hair. Excessive use of elastics in the same place each day can cause breakage.

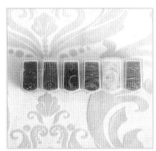

COMBS

We don't use much in the way of brushes at our house. That's not to say brushes are bad, but I have found using combs works best for us. Not every hair type is the same, so it is important to use what gives you the best results and causes the least damage. The following are different combs that I use on a regular basis at our house:

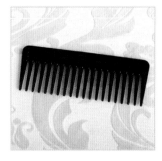

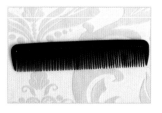

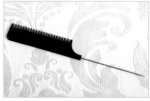

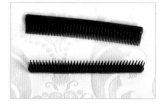

WIDE-TOOTH COMB

In my opinion, these are a must-have. They are wonderful for getting knots out, as well as for combing conditioner through hair in the shower. I bought mine at the dollar store and we have several of them because we use them so much.

BASIC COMB

I also use a basic comb that you can buy anywhere. It has teeth that are closer together on the one end and a bit wider spaced on the other. Once the hair has been detangled with a wide-tooth comb, I use this comb for pretty much every style. Because the teeth are close together they help smooth hair nicely. These types of combs can be purchased anywhere and often come with multiples in a pack.

RAT-TAIL COMB

While this comb can be used for backcombing or teasing hair, I mainly use it for the handle or tail. It is great for tucking in small "bubbles" of hair that poke out or hair that needs to be smoothed. The tail is helpful when parting or sectioning off hair. It's also fantastic to help unravel small braids. (See page 10) I especially like it because the tail is not plastic like a lot of rat-tail combs. Rat-tail combs that are completely plastic with a really tapered handle sometimes have a seam in the plastic that tends to catch and snag the hair. The stainless steel handle/tail doesn't have that issue. These combs can be found at beauty supply stores for a few dollars.

THREE- ROW COMB

This comb is the best comb I've ever found for teasing or backcombing hair. Having three different rows of teeth that are staggered makes all the difference. It's also great for combing out knots and smoothing the top layer of hair after it has been back combed. These can also be purchased at beauty supply stores for a couple dollars.

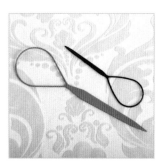

TOPSY TAIL

These are great tools for flipping ponytails and creating a fun new look in your hair. We use them for a few styles in this book. Truth be told, I went for several years without having these, and you can achieve the same flipped ponytail without them. They can be found online, at beauty supply stores or some big box stores carry them. They run about $7 or less.

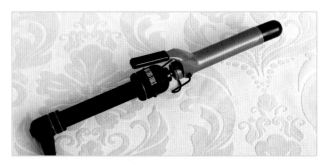

CURLING IRONS & HAIR STRAIGHTENERS

The method most people use to achieve curls is largely determined by how well their hair holds curl. These days there are so many different curling tools out there, but I still just use a few of the basics ones. I normally use a basic 1" barrel curling iron for curls (see above) and I also like curling with my straightener. (aka flat iron.) A curling iron with temperature control is extremely helpful, rather than just one that has high and low settings.

Earlier, I mentioned my old and dying flat iron. I'd been using it for five years to straighten and curl hair, and I even used it in a few of the styles for this book, but as you can see it was on its last leg and

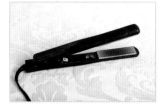

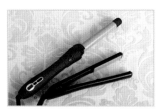

it actually completely broke mid-book! CHI generously hooked me up with some fabulous new tools to help me finish this project. Now I know I said earlier you don't need totally expensive tools to do your hair, and while I still stand by that statement, if you can afford to buy top-of-the-line equipment, by all means, do it! Honestly, it's been nice to have a flat iron and curling iron that tells me how hot they are and that glide through hair so well!

Of course, whenever using heated tools, do so with caution. It takes practice to learn how to use them and you should always use some sort of heat-protecting serum before applying heat (see page 8).

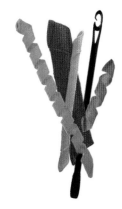

NO HEAT CURLS

On my daughter's hair, I try to use as little heat as possible, but I do like curls in their hair. My favorite way of getting gorgeous curls is to use Curlformers (see page 171).

These are the perfect solution to get amazing curls without heat—especially when I want the entire head curled. They come in several different lengths and thicknesses and they work in any type of hair. Curling with no heat truly saves their hair from damage. They can be slept in, and though it defeats the 'no heat' idea, you can blow them dry to speed up the process. More information about these can be found at www.curlformers.com.

You also can achieve pretty curls without heat, by wrapping sections of your hair around socks or strips of cloth and sleep with them in your hair. Just be sure to do this with fairly dry hair or your hair will still be damp in the morning.

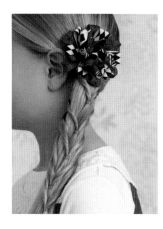

ACCESSORIES

In several of the styles, we have used headbands, flowers, or other accessories. Decorative bobby pins or hairpins, ribbon, or other jewelry are also great ways to dress up a style. These obviously are used to enhance the look of the style, but are optional and are purely based on taste.

STYLING PRODUCTS

THE TYPE OF HAIR you are working with, as well as the style you are trying to achieve, is going to determine what kind of product(s) you will need, and how much of it you will use.

Although it's not technically a styling product, when working with younger girls, spraying the hair with water for braids, twists, etc., is key to getting flawless hairstyles. A gel or mousse of some kind is also extremely helpful in keeping the hair tidy and in place.

Other than water, for styles in this book and on our blog we only use a few basic styling products.

> HAIR SPRAY
>
> HEAT-PROTECTING SERUM OR SPRAY
>
> POMADE OR WAX
>
> MOUSSE

HAIR SPRAY OR FINISHING SPRAY

Spray after you are done with a style to hold things in place. Depending on the style, you may find it helpful to spray sections as you work to cut down on fly-aways or hold something firmly in place.

HEAT-PROTECTING SERUM OR SPRAY

Spray on or rub through areas of hair to protect it when you are curling or straightening. It's also a good idea to put some in your hair when it is wet before you blow it dry. Minimal heat is always best, but unfortunately, sometimes the things that we use to style our hair aren't always best for the health of our hair. So I suggest always using a heat protector.

POMADE OR WAX

There are countless types of these on the market, and most are very similar in what they do. They help hold hair in place and give shine to your hair. Depending on what you need it for, a little can go a long way. I tend to use pomade for small sections of hair in updos that need to be held together, like pin curls.

MOUSSE

I use mousse whenever I plan on putting curlers in hair. It's best to rub it into wet hair to help create body, and it also helps the curls hold longer.

TIPS FOR HEALTHIER HAIR

I'M NOT GOING to pretend I know a lot about every kind of hair type. I can tell you, however, that genes, unfortunately (or fortunately), have a lot to do with the kind of hair you have. Thick or thin, course or fine, straight or curly—it's from your genes.

If you aren't one of those who was blessed to have amazing locks, don't fret. There are things you can do to help your hair along. One major factor that can play into the health of your hair is diet. Believe it or not, what you put into your mouth (or a child's mouth) can be the difference between great healthy hair and "hat day" hair.

It may be obvious, but one big way to help prevent a lot of breakage and damage to your hair is to limit the amount of heat you apply to it. Our hair is most at risk of being damaged when it is wet. If you can get away it, avoid using your hair dryer on a daily basis, but also be sure you aren't rubbing your hair to death with your towel to dry it instead. Gently squeezing your hair is a much better way to go, and by so doing, you can help cut down on frizz and split ends. If you must use heat, be sure to protect your hair with a good heat-protecting serum, cream, or spray.

If you are one who always wears ponytails or puts them in your daughter's hair, constantly using elastics or ponytail holders can also cause breakage. If you must wear ponytails regularly, don't always put them in the same place every time.

One thing I've found that is great for hair is unrefined coconut oil. It can be found in the cooking aisle of most grocery stores. It comes as a solid, but once you rub it in your fingers to warm it up it turns soft and liquefies. It has so many amazing uses and benefits. It can act as a deep conditioner to help damaged hair, it helps fight frizz, and it nourishes the scalp. Some say it helps their hair grow faster and healthier too.

Shampoo and conditioners can also help or hinder your hair. While I'm not one to buy the most expensive brands on the market, I don't recommend buying the cheapest either. Chances are if you are buying a ninety-nice cent bottle of shampoo, don't expect to have amazing results. In the end, it's the ingredients that matter, not necessarily the price. Also remember that what may work for one doesn't always work for another. Trying different products and talking to your stylist about your hair type and what kind of products are best for you is my advice.

OTHER HELPFUL TIPS

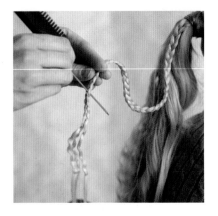

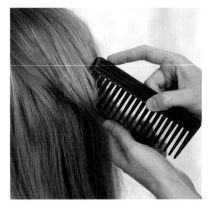

REMOVING BRAIDS

As was mentioned before, when discussing rat-tail combs, a quick way to remove braids, especially micro braids, is to use the end of your rat-tail comb. Starting at the bottom of the braid, simply stick the pointed end of your comb through the braid and gently pull it down the hair until you reach the bottom. Moving up the braid, do a few sections at a time, and you will quickly undo the braid.

DETANGLING HAIR

No matter what you call them, unless your hair is a pixie cut or shorter, chances are you get knots or tangles in your hair. There are so many products out there to help fight the battle, but here are three things that I know help combat knots.

First, as was briefly touched on, invest in a wide-tooth comb that you can keep in your shower. When conditioning your hair, put most of the conditioner in the length of your hair, not up on your scalp. Once you've worked it through your hair, take your wide-tooth comb and comb the conditioner through the length of your hair. Do this until you feel your hair is tangle free. Then as you are rinsing the conditioner out, continue to comb through your hair as well.

Second, when you are working with hair and come upon knots, try turning your comb vertical instead of horizontal. This works especially well with a wide-tooth comb. With one hand, hold the section of hair with the knot, and with the other hand turn the comb vertical. Holding the hair above the knotted area as you comb can also be a way to prevent a bit of discomfort when combing. You are "picking" through the knotted section with just a few teeth of the comb, instead of dragging the entire comb through the section, which sometimes can make more knots.

And third, if you or your daughter tend to have excessive knots or look like you have a rats nest in your hair when you wake up in the morning, invest in a silk pillowcase. It's been a well-kept secret by stylists and movie stars for ages that silk pillowcases are gentler on your hair (and also kinder to your skin). Not only are they better for your skin and help cut down on knots in your hair, there's another benefit as well. Come morning, depending on how you style your hair, you may find your hair hasn't changed a whole lot from the night before. This can be a huge time saver in the morning, especially if you're running late and don't have time to do much with your hair!

BOBBY PIN TIPS/TRICKS

If you try to hold back a small section of hair and find your bobby pin slips, you can do a couple things. Try using two of them to form an X (see below).

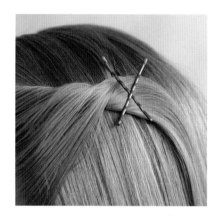

It's also been said that the wavy side of a bobby pin is actually supposed to lay on your scalp and the flat side should face up for a better hold. Try it out and see which works better for you.

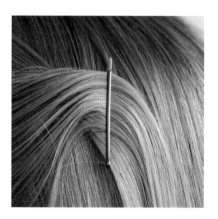

Another way to get those bobby pins to stay put is by laying bobby pins out on a paper towel and misting them with hair spray. The hair spray will give them a stickier surface, which should keep them from sliding out of your hair.

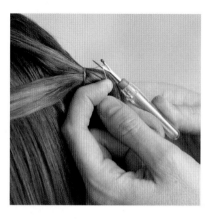

REMOVING ELASTICS

When removing elastics from a hairstyle, try not to pull them down and out of the hair. This can cause breakage, and often times creates knots. Instead, carefully take a seam ripper/unpicker, a pair of finger nail clippers, or if you are extremely cautious, use a small pair of scissors to cut one small section of the elastic. Once it is snipped, simply unwind the elastic from around the hair, helping prevent knots and unwanted damage to the hair.

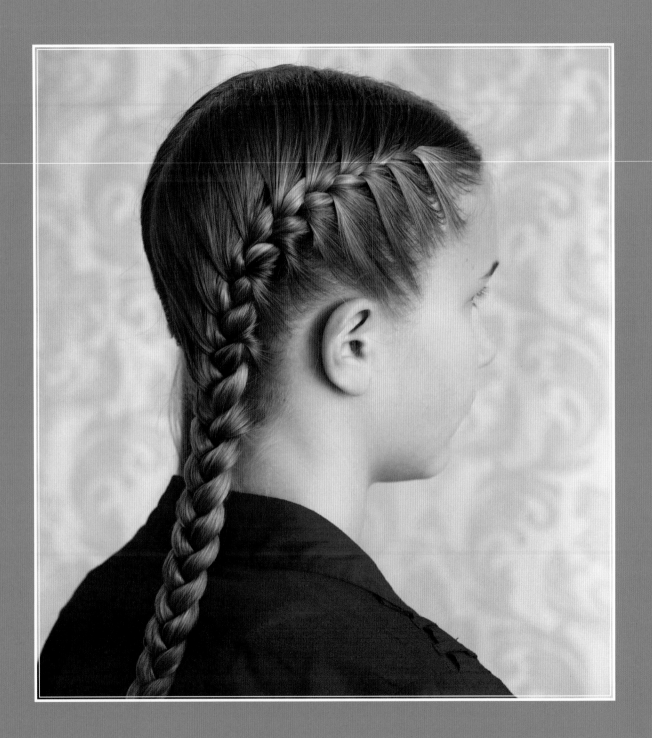

CHAPTER 2
The Basic Techniques

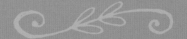

The Basic Techniques

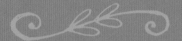

Master the basics and you will be able to create hundreds of different hairstyles by combining them and making up your own creative styles.

WHILE MANY people know how to do basic hair techniques, many do not. Years ago when looking for books or websites, it frustrated me to find things that were only final images of hairstyles and didn't show the step-by-steps of how the hairstyle was created or I'd find tons of words describing something but no pictures. Because of that, this book includes many of my favorite techniques at the beginning for you and all the hairstyles are step-by-step pictures and instructions. To some, what I'm sharing in this section may seem extremely basic, but over the years, so many people have told me that it is with these basics that they struggle. I'm a strong believer that if you know a lot of basic hair techniques you then have the skills to create countless hairstyles.

If you struggle with a specific technique, do it over and over again until you master it! When my daughters were smaller, didn't have as much hair, or were napping, I'd practice on a doll head I bought, that in theory was supposed to be a toy! That's how I mastered certain techniques. It just depends on how determined you are to learn something.

If you are new to "doing hair" I'd suggest trying to braid or twist hair that is slightly damp. I find it makes the hair a little easier to manage. Depending on the hairstyle and look you want to achieve, damp hair sometimes works best. If you prefer to work with dry hair and are worried about things not looking "perfect"— you're in luck. These days, "messy" is the style (even with updos sometimes), so most likely, no one will give it a second thought.

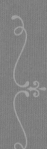

TWISTS

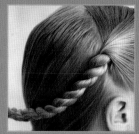
ROPE BRAID/TWIST
16

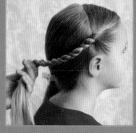
UNEVEN ROPE
BRAID/TWIST
17

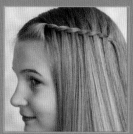
WATERFALL TWIST
18

BRAIDS

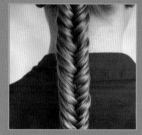
FISHBONE BRAID
20

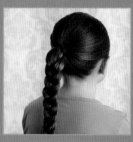
3-STRAND BRAID
22

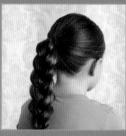
PANCAKE BRAID
23

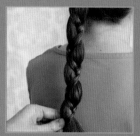
UNEVEN
3-STRAND BRAID
25

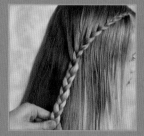
LACE BRAID (ONE-SIDED
OR HALF-FRENCH BRAID)
26

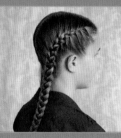
FRENCH BRAID
28

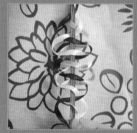
4-STRAND BRAID
(DEMONSTRATED WITH RIBBON)
30

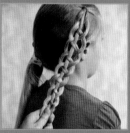
4-STRAND BRAID
32

PONYTAILS,
BUNS & MORE

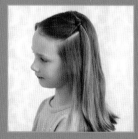
FLIPPED PONYTAIL
34

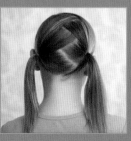
PARTS & PONYTAILS
35

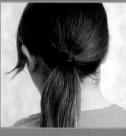
HAIR-WRAPPED
PONYTAIL
36

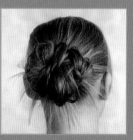
EASY MESSY BUN
38

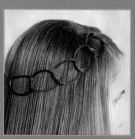
HAIR CHAINS
40

ROPE BRAID/TWIST

If you are new at making a rope braid, you might find it easier to start with a ponytail secured by an elastic. They can be made anywhere on the head, with or without the start of a ponytail.

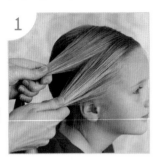
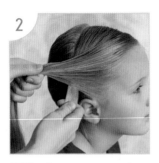
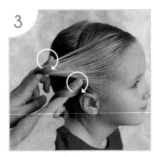
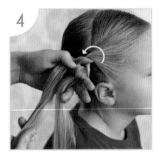

STEP 1 Take a section of hair and divide it into two even sections.

STEP 2 Cross the right (or bottom section as shown in the picture) over the left (or top) section of hair so it makes an X.

STEP 3 Twist both sections of hair to the right (clockwise). In the beginning, you may find it easier to wrap the hair around your fingers to twist.

STEP 4 Then pass the right strand (bottom strand) over the left strand (top strand) in a counterclockwise direction. You may need to momentarily hold both sections of hair with your left hand when the sections have traded places to prevent it from untwisting (as shown). Then pass the right strand back to your right hand to start twisting again.

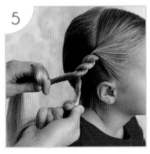

STEP 5 Repeat steps 2–4 as many times as needed until you reach the desired length of twist. Secure the end with an elastic or clip.

NOTE: The rope braid may loosen and unwind slightly, but this is normal. The tighter you make it, the tighter it will stay once the end is tied off.

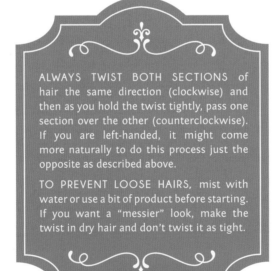

ALWAYS TWIST BOTH SECTIONS of hair the same direction (clockwise) and then as you hold the twist tightly, pass one section over the other (counterclockwise). If you are left-handed, it might come more naturally to do this process just the opposite as described above.

TO PREVENT LOOSE HAIRS, mist with water or use a bit of product before starting. If you want a "messier" look, make the twist in dry hair and don't twist it as tight.

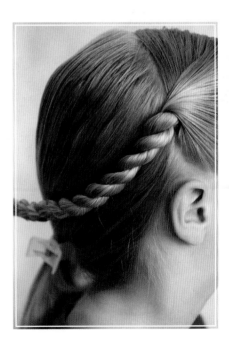

TWISTS

UNEVEN ROPE BRAID/TWIST

The process for this twist is exactly the same as a regular rope braid shown on the previous page, except you do not use even amounts of hair.

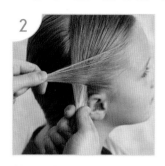

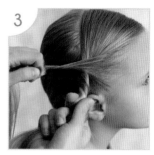

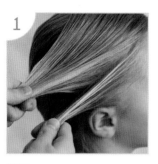

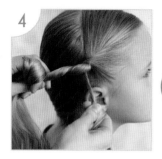

STEP 1 Take a section of hair and divide it into two **uneven** sections. The left section should be thick; the right section should be thin.

STEP 2 Cross the thinner section of hair over the thicker section of hair so they trade places, making an X.

STEP 3 Twist both sections of hair to the right (clockwise).

STEP 4 Then pass the right, thicker section over the left, thinner section to the left (counterclockwise) so they trade places. Be sure to hold the hair tightly so it doesn't untwist.

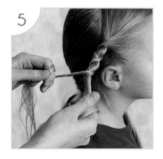

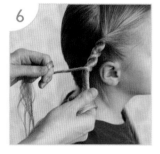

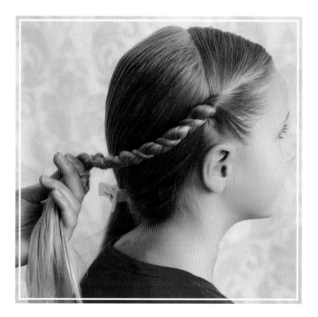

STEP 5 Repeat steps 3–4.

STEP 6 Continue twisting until you reach the desired length and look of the twist. Secure the end with an elastic or clip.

NOTE: The rope braid will possibly unwind and loosen up slightly, but this is normal. The tighter you make it, the tighter it will stay once the end is tied off.

TWISTS

17

WATERFALL TWIST

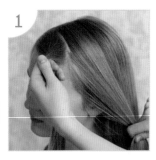

STEP 1 Make a part on the top of the head. Then section out a small piece of hair along the hairline at the top of the forehead.

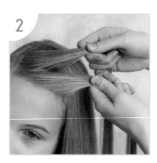

STEP 2 Divide the section of hair into 2 pieces.

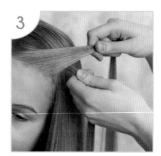

STEP 3 Cross the left piece (bottom) over the right piece (top), creating an X.

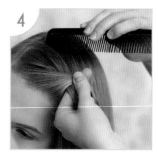

STEP 4 Hold that section of hair in one hand and, using a comb or your fingers, grab a small amount of hair just behind the hair you crossed over.

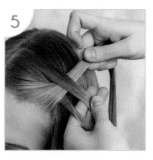

STEP 5 Smooth out that section of hair and lay it on top of the piece you crossed over in step 3.

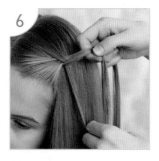

STEP 6 Let the piece from step 4 hang down into the rest of the hair. Then cross the bottom piece over the top piece. You will be working with these same two strands of hair for the entire twist. You never drop them.

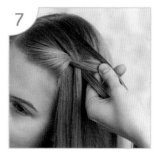

STEP 7 Grab another small section of hair and lay it over (or in between) the original pieces from step 3.

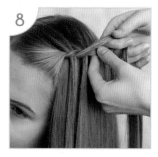

STEP 8 Repeat the process, letting this small section of hair hang down with the rest of the hair. Pass the bottom piece over the top piece.

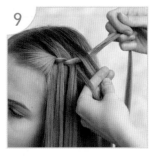

STEP 9 Continue this process, grabbing small sections and laying them between the two pieces of hair.

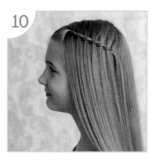

STEP 10 Continue as far as desired and then secure the end with an elastic or a couple bobby pins.

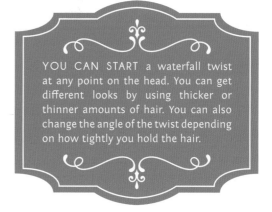

YOU CAN START a waterfall twist at any point on the head. You can get different looks by using thicker or thinner amounts of hair. You can also change the angle of the twist depending on how tightly you hold the hair.

TWISTS

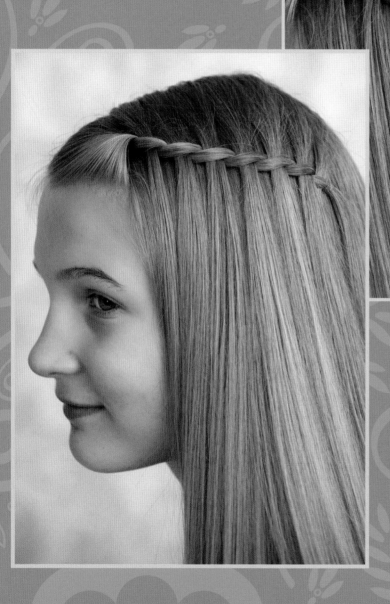

FISHBONE BRAID

This kind of braid can be called different things such as fishtail braid or herringbone braid. No matter what you call it, it is a braid that only uses two strands and crosses small sections back and forth. It's easier than you think, so give it a try!

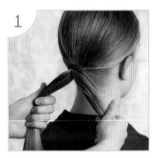

STEP 1 Make a ponytail and divide the hair into two pieces so you have left and right sections.

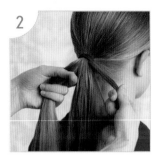

STEP 2 Divide out a small section of hair from the far right side of the section on the right.

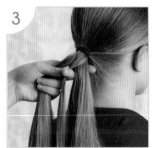

STEP 3 Draw that small section over to the left side and incorporate it into the section on the left.

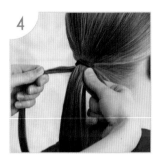

STEP 4 Divide out a small section of hair from the far left side of the section on the left. You may have to hold the piece of hair from step 3 in place with your right hand's thumb.

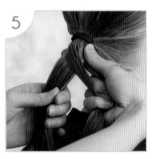

STEP 5 Draw that small section over to the right side and incorporate it into the section on the right. Those small sections that have been passed to each side now form an X and you have completed one full "rotation" of a fishbone braid.

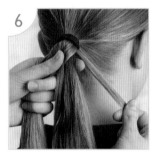

STEP 6 Repeat the steps again, taking a small section from the outer edge of the section on the right.

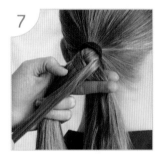

STEP 7 Add it to the hair on the left.

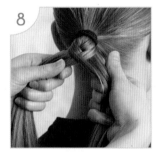

STEP 8 Again on the left side take a small section of hair and pass it to the right side to finish another X.

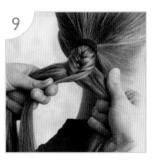

STEP 9 Continue the process of passing a small section from the right over to the left side, and a small section from the left over to the right side.

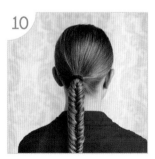

STEP 10 Braid down as far as desired and secure the end with an elastic.

IF YOU ARE NEW at making a fishbone braid, you might have a hard time keeping the braid from sliding, so you may find it easier to start with a ponytail as your base. Once you are more comfortable with this technique, a ponytail is optional. The smaller the sections you pass from side to side, the more intricate of a look you will achieve. You can gain a whole different look depending on if you hold the hair tight or loose, or if you pull on the edges to pancake it.

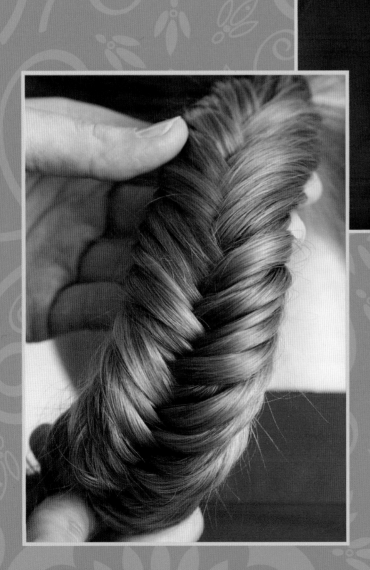

21

3-STRAND BRAID

Braids have been around forever and can be used countless ways to achieve so many different looks. To show the basic technique, the braid is being started from a ponytail.

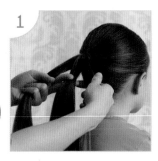

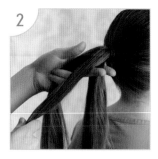

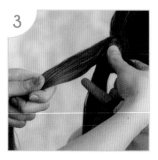

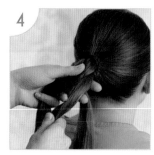

STEP 1 Divide the hair into 3 even sections.

STEP 2 Cross the right section of hair over the middle section so they change places.

STEP 3 Cross the left section of hair over the middle section so it is now in the middle. You have now done one full "rotation" of a braid.

STEP 4 Repeat steps 2–3, crossing the right section over the middle, and then the left section over the middle.

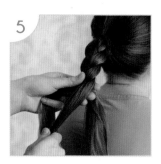

STEP 5 Braid down as far as desired and secure with an elastic.

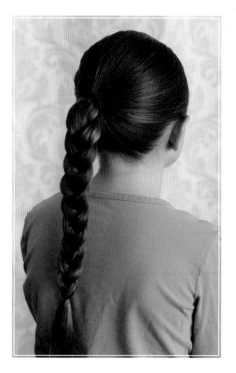

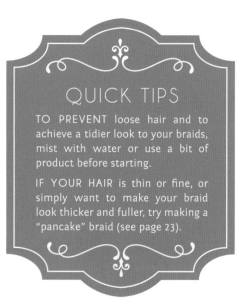

QUICK TIPS

TO PREVENT loose hair and to achieve a tidier look to your braids, mist with water or use a bit of product before starting.

IF YOUR HAIR is thin or fine, or simply want to make your braid look thicker and fuller, try making a "pancake" braid (see page 23).

BRAIDS

22

PANCAKE BRAID

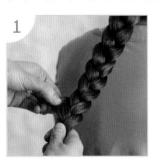

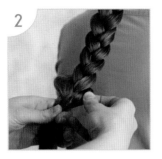

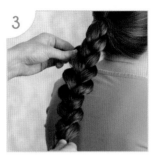

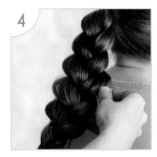

STEP 1 Create a regular 3-strand braid (see page 22). It is a lot easier to do this if the braid is **not** secured at the base with an elastic. Gently hold the braid and, starting at the bottom of the braid, gently tug on the outside edges of the braid.

STEP 2 Work from one side to the other, gently tugging on the outside edge to loosen things up.

STEP 3 Continue working your way up the braid, tugging on the left and ride sides of the braid. Once you reach the top of the braid, you may need to go back and adjust different sections of the braid to even things out.

STEP 4 The more you pull on the edges, the wider and flatter it will become. If you are working with dry hair, you can achieve an even "messier" look by doing this. Secure the end with an elastic once you have achieved the desired look. If I had continued to pull on the braid, it could have been made even wider and flatter.

THE BASIC TECHNIQUES

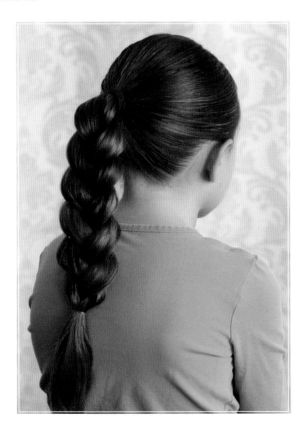

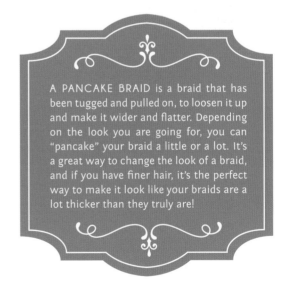

A PANCAKE BRAID is a braid that has been tugged and pulled on, to loosen it up and make it wider and flatter. Depending on the look you are going for, you can "pancake" your braid a little or a lot. It's a great way to change the look of a braid, and if you have finer hair, it's the perfect way to make it look like your braids are a lot thicker than they truly are!

BRAIDS

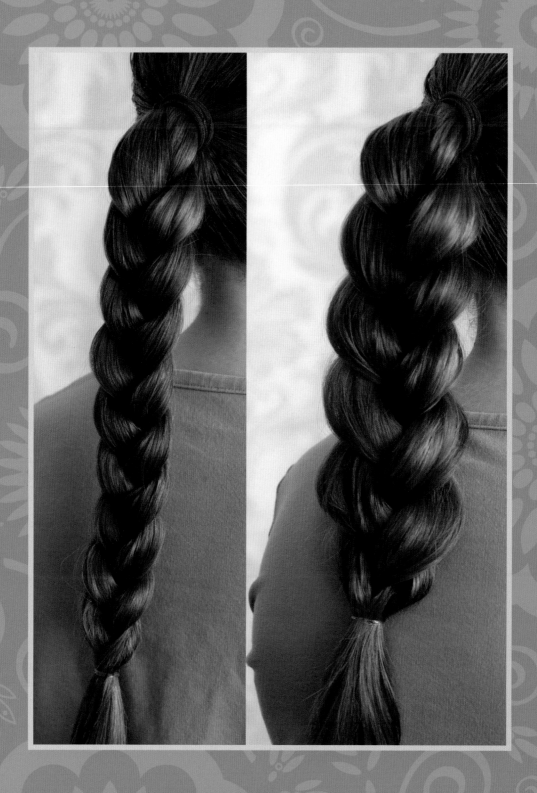

UNEVEN 3-STRAND BRAID

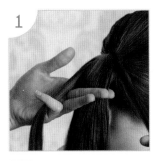

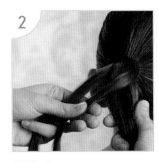

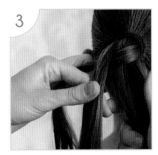

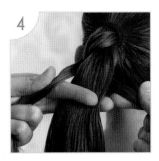

STEP 1 Divide the hair into three sections. The two outside strands should be thin, and the middle section should be thick.

STEP 2 This is done just like a regular 3-strand braid (see page 22) except you have different thicknesses of hair. Cross the far right thin strand over the thick middle strand.

STEP 3 Cross the far left thin strand over the middle strand (which is now the other thin section.) This is one full "rotation" of the braid.

STEP 4 Cross the far right thick strand over the thin middle strand so it ends up back in the middle.

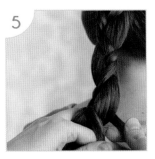

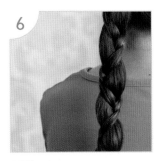

STEP 5 Continue the process of crossing the right strand over the middle strand and left strand over the middle strand.

STEP 6 Braid down as far as you wish and secure the end with an elastic. Using uneven sections gives the braid a very pretty and unique look.

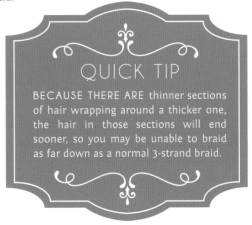

QUICK TIP

BECAUSE THERE ARE thinner sections of hair wrapping around a thicker one, the hair in those sections will end sooner, so you may be unable to braid as far down as a normal 3-strand braid.

BONUS STYLE

ADDITIONAL LOOK for uneven 3-strand braid

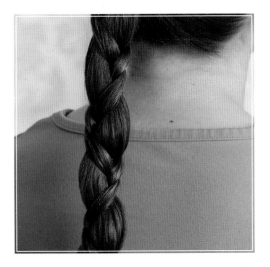

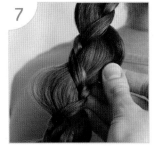

STEP 7 If you wish to give the uneven 3-strand braid an even more unique look, you can pancake it by gently pulling on the thicker sections of the braid, working up each side of the braid. This can be done as much or as little as you like depending on the desired look you wish to achieve.

LACE BRAID (ONE-SIDED OR HALF-FRENCH BRAID)

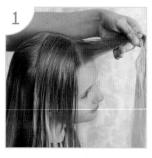

STEP 1 Part the hair on the left from the forehead to the crown. Then make a small triangular part, sectioning out a small amount of hair.

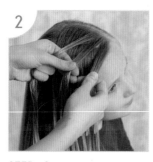

STEP 2 Divide the hair into three sections.

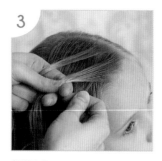

STEP 3 Cross the right (bottom) section of hair over the middle strand.

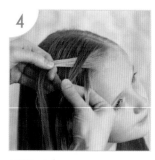

STEP 4 Cross the left (top) section of hair over the middle strand.

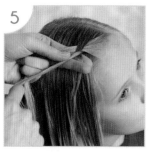

STEP 5 Repeat the process, and cross the right (bottom) section over the middle section.

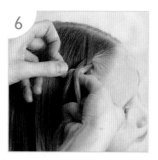

STEP 6 Cross the left (top) section over the middle section so it now becomes the middle section and stop.

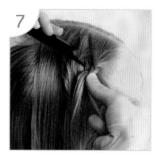

STEP 7 With a comb or your fingers, grab a small amount of hair from above the braid.

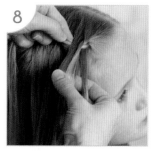

STEP 8 Add that hair to the middle section, incorporating it into the hair you crossed over in step 6.

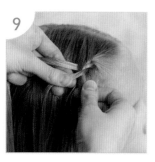

STEP 9 Cross the right section (bottom) over the middle section. Do not add hair to this section.

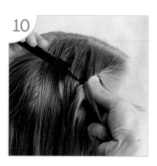

STEP 10 Again cross the left section over to the middle, and add hair from above. Then cross right over without adding hair.

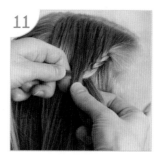

STEP 11 Continue repeating steps 6–9 as many times as desired.

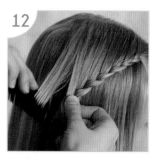

STEP 12 Once you reach the crown, you can stop adding hair to the left side if you like. Continue braiding the hair, making a regular 3-strand braid, and do not add hair any longer. Braid as far down as desired, and secure with an elastic.

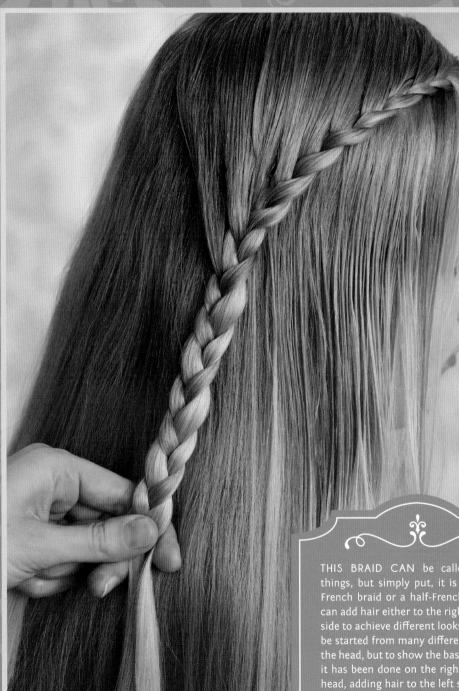

THIS BRAID CAN be called different things, but simply put, it is a one-sided French braid or a half-French braid. You can add hair either to the right or the left side to achieve different looks. It can also be started from many different points on the head, but to show the basic technique it has been done on the right side of the head, adding hair to the left side.

27

FRENCH BRAID

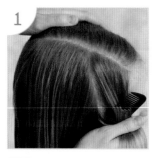

STEP 1 Part out a small section of hair.

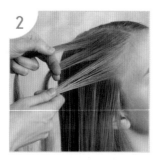

STEP 2 Divide that section into three pieces like you would a regular 3-strand braid.

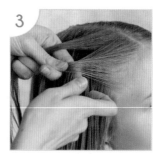

STEP 3 Pass the right (or bottom) section over the middle section so they trade places.

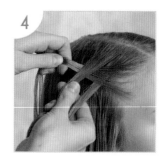

STEP 4 Pass the left (or top) section over the new middle section so they trade places.

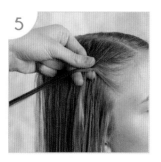

STEP 5 Pass the right (or bottom) section over the middle section.

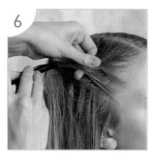

STEP 6 With a comb or your fingers, grab a small section of the loose hair on the right side of the braid. Add it to the hair that was just passed to the middle section.

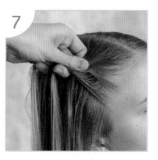

STEP 7 It may be necessary to smooth the section of hair that was just added to the braid so it is free of bumps or tangles.

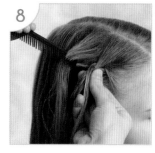

STEP 8 Pass the left (or top) section over the middle section. Then with a comb or your fingers, grab a small section of the loose hair on the left side of the braid and add it to the hair that was just passed to the middle section.

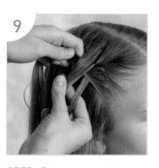

STEP 9 This is one full "rotation" of a French braid. You have now added hair from both the left and the right sides to the braid one time. At this point, two sections will be thicker from adding hair. The section on the far right will still be thin because no hair has been added to it yet.

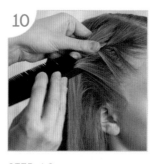

STEP 10 Repeat the steps 5–9, passing the right section over to the middle, and then add hair to it. Then pass the left section over the middle, and add hair to it.

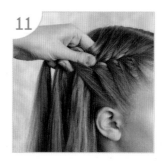

STEP 11 Continue braiding as far as desired. To keep the braid nice and tight, pinch the hair close to the hair with which you are working.

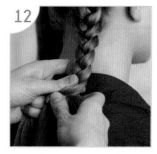

STEP 12 Once you run out of hair to add, or no longer wish to add hair, continue making a regular 3-strand braid and secure the end with an elastic. If desired, gently use a comb to smooth out any bumps or gaps in the hair.

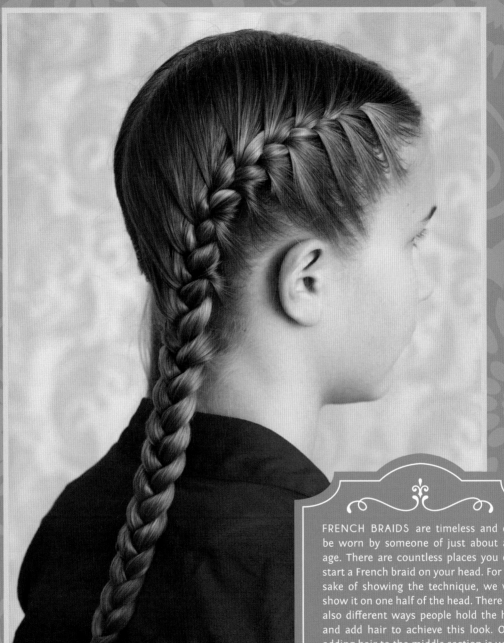

FRENCH BRAIDS are timeless and can be worn by someone of just about any age. There are countless places you can start a French braid on your head. For the sake of showing the technique, we will show it on one half of the head. There are also different ways people hold the hair and add hair to achieve this look. Only adding hair to the middle section is what is easiest for me. This French braid was done in fairly damp hair to make it a neat and tidy braid.

4-STRAND BRAID (DEMONSTRATED WITH RIBBON)

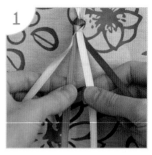

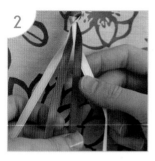

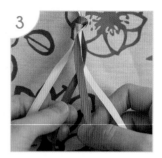

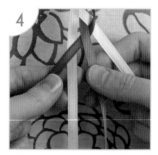

STEP 1 Start with four sections. From left to right—light purple, pink, white, and dark purple.

STEP 2 Start on the right side. Cross the dark purple over the white ribbon.

STEP 3 Then pass the dark purple under the pink ribbon. The purple has just gone "over and under."

STEP 4 Now you will work from the left side. Cross the light purple under the dark purple ribbon.

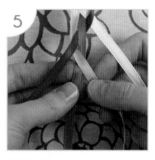

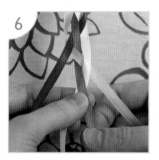

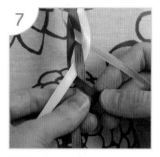

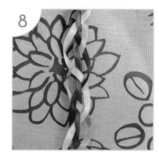

STEP 5 Cross the light purple over the pink ribbon. The light purple has just gone "under and over." This is one full "rotation" of the braid from both the right and left sides. Now the white ribbon is on the far right and you will start weaving with it in the next step.

STEP 6 Now you start again. You always weave with the outermost strand—regardless of its color. Cross the white ribbon over the light purple and under the pink. Dark purple is on the far left and you will start weaving with it in the next step.

STEP 7 Cross the dark purple under the white and over the pink. This is a second full rotation of the braid. From here you would start on the right side again and cross the light purple over the dark purple and under the pink.

STEP 8 Continue the pattern of taking the outer right strand "over and under" and then the outer left strand "under and over." This will make a 4-strand braid. Notice the pink strand runs right down the center of the braid.

BONUS STYLE

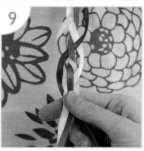

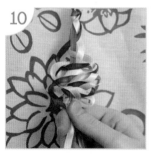

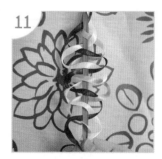

STEP 9 If you braided correctly, the pink strand should always be in the middle position (either the 2nd or 3rd strand of the braid) Take the pink ribbon in one hand and hold it tight and gently push up the other ribbons.

STEP 10 Continue pushing the other ribbons upward so the other strands bunch together.

STEP 11 Then gently pull them back down and you will have an intricate design that loops around the pink ribbon. It looks totally amazing in hair when you create this 4-strand slide braid!

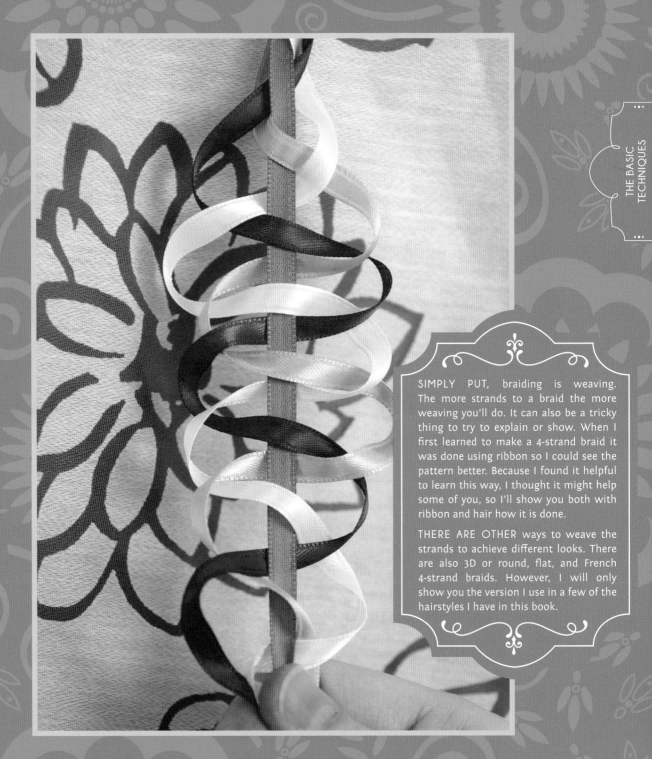

SIMPLY PUT, braiding is weaving. The more strands to a braid the more weaving you'll do. It can also be a tricky thing to try to explain or show. When I first learned to make a 4-strand braid it was done using ribbon so I could see the pattern better. Because I found it helpful to learn this way, I thought it might help some of you, so I'll show you both with ribbon and hair how it is done.

THERE ARE OTHER ways to weave the strands to achieve different looks. There are also 3D or round, flat, and French 4-strand braids. However, I will only show you the version I use in a few of the hairstyles I have in this book.

4-STRAND BRAID

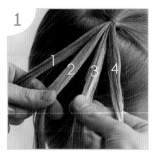

STEP 1 Divide the hair into four even sections.

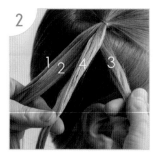

STEP 2 Begin on the far right using strand #4. Cross strand #4 over strand #3.

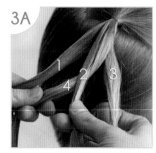

STEP 3A Cross strand #4 under strand #2.

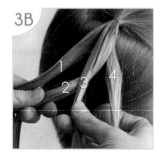

STEP 3B Now the numbers reset since the original strand #4 is now in the #2 position.

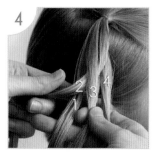

STEP 4 Cross strand #1 under strand #2.

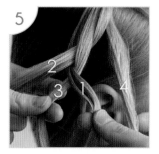

STEP 5 Cross strand #1 over strand #3. This is one full rotation of the braid from both sides.

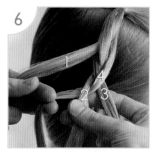

STEP 6 Now you will start the pattern over again. Start back on the right side. In this picture strand #4 on the far right has gone over strand #3 and under strand #2.

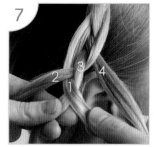

STEP 7 And back to the left side, strand #1 has gone under strand #2 and over strand #3, completing another full rotation of the braid.

BONUS STYLE

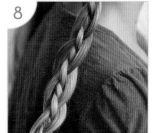

STEP 8 Continue the pattern to create the braid. Regardless of strand number—the pattern always remains the same. Always weave with the outermost strand. Take that outer right strand and cross it "over and then under." Then take the outer left strand and cross it "under and then over."

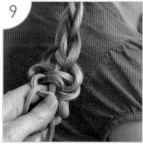

STEP 9 As shown with the ribbon tutorial, you can also create a 4-strand slide up braid. After you have completed braiding, find the strand that runs right down the middle of the braid. It should be in the second or third position of the braid. While holding that strand with one hand, push the other strands up toward the scalp.

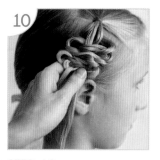

STEP 10 Push them up completely until they are bunched together at the top. Continue holding the one strand while slowly sliding the sections back down.

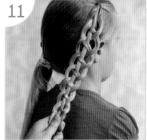

STEP 11 This creates an amazing new look to your braid. You can pull on the edges further if you desire to make the circles all uniform in size and shape. Regardless of if you create the slide-up 4-strand look or the regular 4-strand look from step 8, this braid is always a perfect touch to any hairstyle!

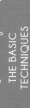

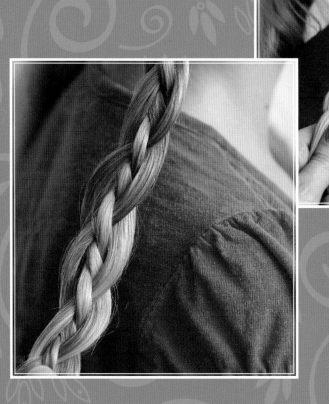

IF YOU ARE NEW to 4-strand braiding, you might find it helpful to check out the step-by-steps using ribbon on the previous page. You also may find it helpful to begin with a ponytail as a base and use hair that is fairly damp to prevent fly-aways. These can be done in big or small amounts of hair for different looks.

TO TRY TO HELP make things less confusing I've numbered the strands 1–4 from left to right. Because I'm right handed, starting from the right is more natural for me. If you are left handed, you can reverse the order and things will work the same.

FLIPPED PONYTAIL

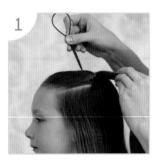

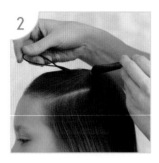

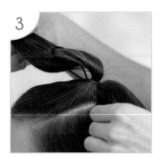

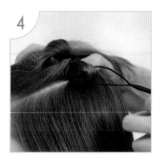

STEP 1 Make a ponytail and position the pointed end of the Topsy Tail toward the hair elastic. Be sure the ponytail isn't too tight or it will make it difficult to do this technique.

STEP 2 Insert the pointed end through the center of the ponytail so it is under the hair elastic and on the scalp.

STEP 3 Place your fingers through the looped end of the Topsy Tail and pull the end of the ponytail through the loop.

STEP 4 Gently begin to pull on the pointed end of the Topsy Tail with one hand. Keep holding the end of the ponytail with the other hand so it does not come out of the looped end of the Topsy Tail. Continue pulling on the pointed end of the Topsy Tail until the entire ponytail has been pulled underneath the hair elastic and the ponytail has "flipped."

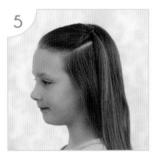

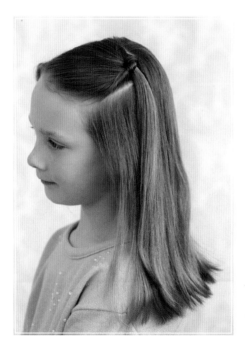

STEP 5 Smooth out the ponytail with a comb once you have flipped it under the elastic.

PONYTAILS, BUNS & MORE

QUICK TIPS

THESE CAN BE called many different names: flipped ponytails, topsy tails, pull throughs, knots . . . but no matter what you call them, they are versatile and girls of all ages use them in hairstyles. You can use big or small amounts of hair, and you can do them anywhere on the head. You just need a ponytail to start. The tool being used is called a Topsy Tail and can be found at most beauty supply stores or online.

THIS TECHNIQUE can still be done even if you don't have a Topsy Tail. Simply loosen the ponytail slightly and with the end of your rat-tail comb or with your fingers, make an hole in the hair against the scalp below the elastic. Tuck the ponytail through with your fingers and pull the ends out the other side.

PARTS & PONYTAILS

A common complaint I hear from people is that they can't make a part that is straight. I'll admit getting a part to be straight does come with practice, but if it's something you just can't seem to get down, then try making a part that is zigzagged or wavy. As in—don't make a straight part on purpose!

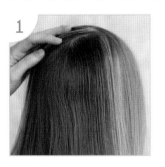

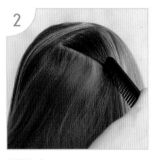

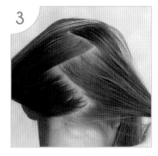

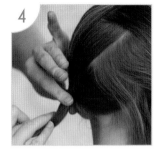

STEP 1 With your comb, or tail of a rat-tail comb, "draw" through the hair on the back of the head. Angle the part off to the left a couple inches.

STEP 2 Then branch off of that part to the right at an angle.

STEP 3 Continue down the back of the head. You can make the zigzag as close together or as far apart as desired.

STEP 4 Gather all the hair on the left side of the part into a ponytail and secure with an elastic. Repeat on the right side of the head as well.

5A

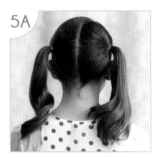

5B

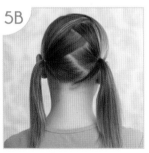

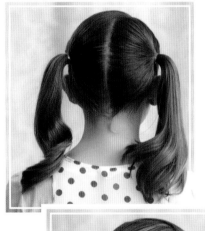

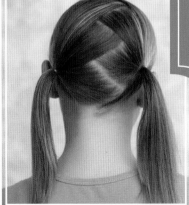

STEP 5A & 5B While a straight part down the middle of the head is always nice. A zigzag part is always more fun and playful!

QUICK TIPS

IF YOU TAKE the tip of your rat-tail comb almost like you are "drawing" on the scalp and go back and forth in a zigzag pattern, you can create a great part. To achieve different looks you can make the zigzag pattern as big and wide or thin and small as you like. Anywhere a straight part is called for you can always substitute it with a zigzag part if you prefer.

ZIGZAG PARTS are great for helping align the ponytails evenly on one side of the head to the other.

PONYTAILS, BUNS & MORE

35

HAIR-WRAPPED PONYTAIL

This technique is great when you don't want your elastic to show or if you don't have a fun accessory to cover the elastic.

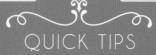

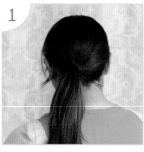

1

STEP 1 Gather desired amount of hair and make a ponytail. Secure with a ponytail holder or elastic.

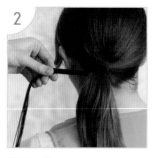

2

STEP 2 Draw out a small section of hair from underneath the ponytail and mist with water or hair spray. Comb the section to smooth it out.

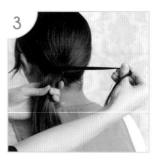

3

STEP 3 Draw the small section of hair over the base of the ponytail to the right, covering the ponytail holder.

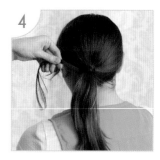

4

STEP 4 Wrapping in a clockwise direction, bring the small section of hair underneath the pony and back out the other side. Wrap as many times as needed, or until you almost run out of hair and the ponytail holder is covered.

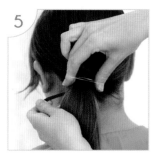

5

STEP 5 With a small clear elastic (we used a colored one so you can see the process better), place the elastic right next to the edge of the wrapped hair. With your other hand, be sure to keep holding onto the small section of hair under the ponytail.

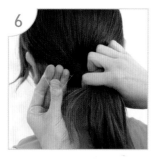

6

STEP 6 Wrap the clear elastic around the ponytail, being sure to include the small section from below.

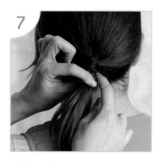

7

STEP 7 Continue wrapping the elastic so it is as close to the wrapped hair as possible, until the elastic is nice and tight.

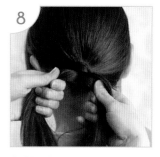

8

STEP 8 If the elastic shows slightly, simply divide the ponytail in half and cinch it to push the elastic up under the wrapped hair.

QUICK TIPS

THIS TECHNIQUE can also be done using a bobby pin to secure the wrapped hair, but often times the bobby pin shows or slides out. Using an elastic to secure the wrapped hair solves that problem!

ONCE THE ponytail holder is covered, stop wrapping so the small section of hair is on the underside of the ponytail.

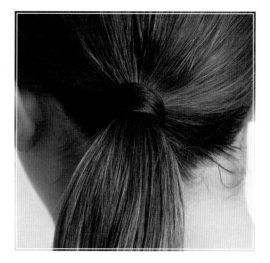

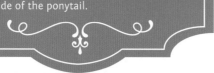

PONYTAILS, BUNS & MORE

THE BASIC TECHNIQUES

36

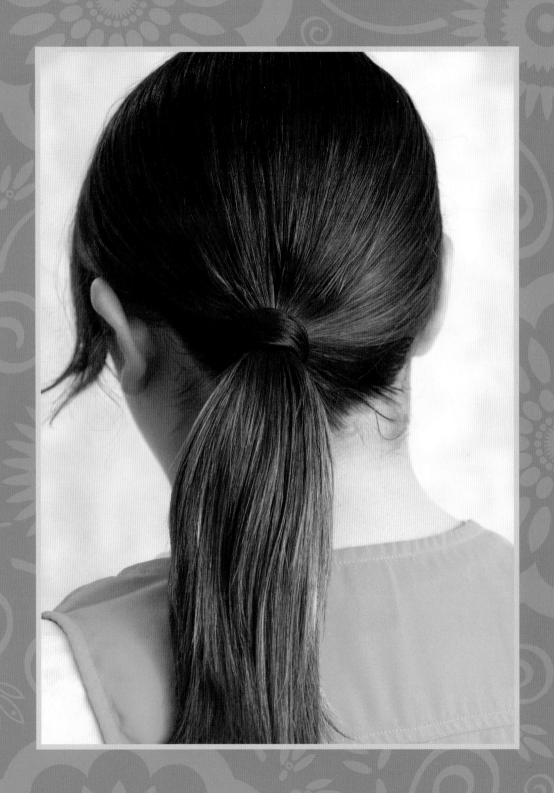

EASY MESSY BUN

This works best with wet or damp hair. If you want an even messier look, use dry hair.

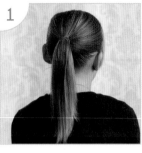

STEP 1 Gather hair into a pony-tail and secure with a ponytail holder.

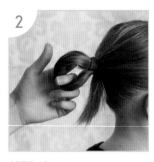

STEP 2 Wrap a second elastic around the base of the ponytail like you are going to make another ponytail. On the last wrap of the elastic, do not pull the ponytail all the way through. Leave the pony-tail in a loop with the ends poking out underneath.

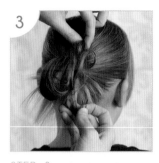

STEP 3 To break up the loop, pinch a small section of hair from the loop and pull it upward and pinch a small section of hair from the loop and pull it down.

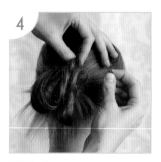

STEP 4 Secure the section you pulled up with a bobby pin to the back of the head.

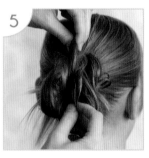

STEP 5 Moving to the left, repeat the same motion, pinching a bit of hair and pulling it up, and pinching hair and pulling it down.

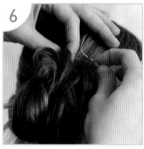

STEP 6 Secure the top section with another bobby pin.

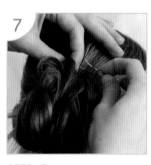

STEP 7 Repeat as many times as needed to pull apart the loop and give it a messier look. Pinch and pull sections as desired and secure with bobby pins so the bun is shaped nicely and there are no gaps between the bun and head. Secure hair under the bun with bobby pins if needed.

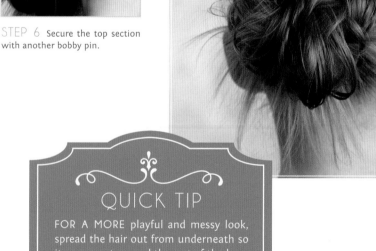

QUICK TIP

FOR A MORE playful and messy look, spread the hair out from underneath so it sprays out around the rest of the bun.

PONYTAILS, BUNS & MORE

BONUS STYLE
FOR A "TIDIER" messy bun

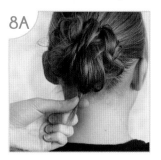

8A

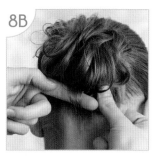

8B

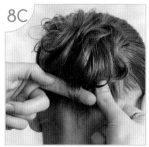

8C

STEP 8A For a less messy look, gather all the loose ends that stuck out around the bun.

STEP 8B Wrap the hair around your finger to loop under the bun.

STEP 8C Tuck the ends up to hide them, and secure with a bobby pin.

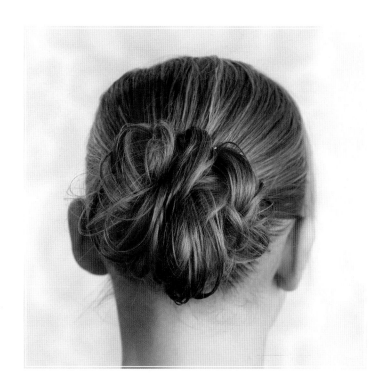

PONYTAILS, BUNS & MORE

HAIR CHAINS

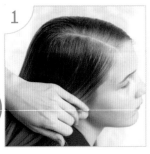

STEP 1 These chains can be done anywhere on the head, but starting at the hairline or from a part is recommended. To demonstrate the technique a side part has been made and the chain will be started from that point.

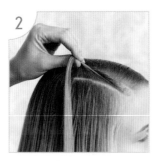

STEP 2 Section out a very small amount of hair parallel to the part. The smaller the section, the thinner the chain will be.

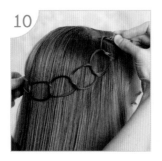

STEP 3 Divide the section of hair in two pieces.

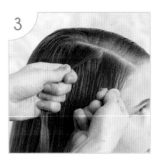

STEP 4 Cross the right piece over the left piece, then pass it under the left piece and up through the hole. This step is like the first step of tying a shoe.

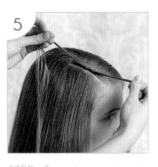

STEP 5 Pull on both ends, cinching the hair so it pulls tight and lays on the scalp.

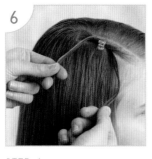

STEP 6 Place a tiny claw clip in the middle of the knot to ensure it does not loosen.

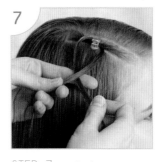

STEP 7 With the two pieces of hair cross the right piece over the left, then pass it under the left piece and up through the hole.

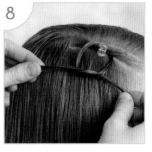

STEP 8 This time, do not pull the hair tight. Only pull on the ends until it forms a circle of hair, or a "link" in the chain. Gently pull on the ends until the link reaches the desired size.

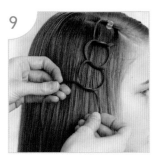

STEP 9 Continue to repeat the above steps adding links to the chain. These can be as big or small as you would like.

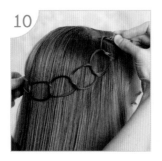

STEP 10 Once the chain is as long as desired and the end is secured, remove the tiny claw clip from the start of the chain. Spray the finished chain with hair spray to ensure it keeps its shape and definition.

TO ACHIEVE a flawless look with this technique, very damp hair, or hair treated with product is recommended. A gentle hand is also needed when creating them. If anchoring into a ponytail or another part of a hairstyle, do not pull the chain too tight or the links will lose the circular shape. They are meant to be draped over or gently placed on top of other hair so they stand out.

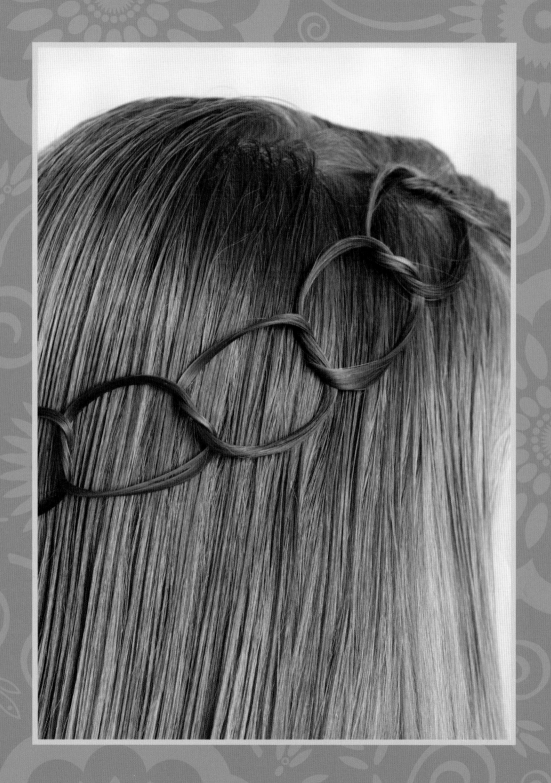

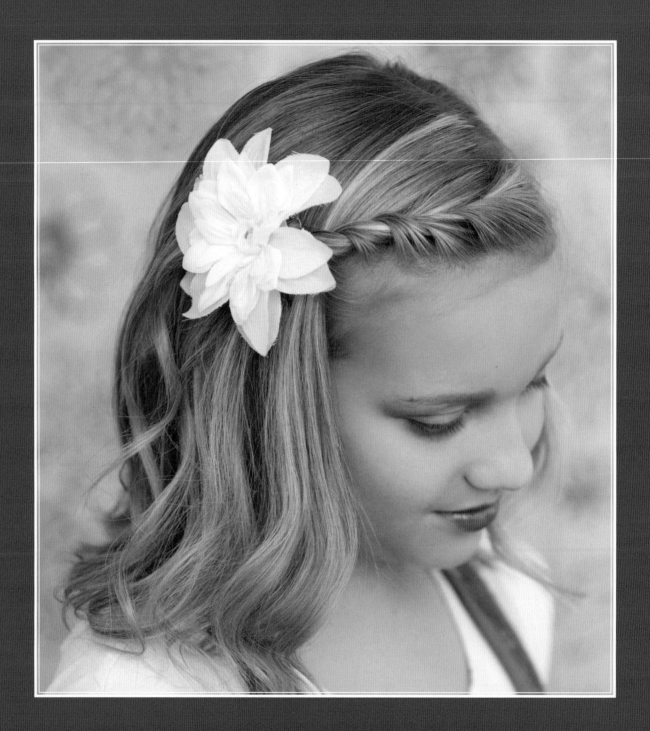

CHAPTER 3
Easy & Effortless Styles

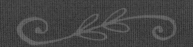

Easy & Effortless Styles

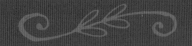

*Simple styles for the beginner or when you just need
to get out the door quickly in the morning.*

THESE STYLES are perfect for the beginner or if you're just in a hurry to get out the door in the morning. They are intended to incorporate techniques that are not too difficult or that require much time. Everyone works with hair at a different speed and skill level, so some of these may take longer than others. I wanted to share styles that were more than pigtails or braids, which are easy, quick, and pleasing to the eye. The hope is that the more you practice the techniques in the last, chapter the styles in the next chapters will become easy and effortless as well!

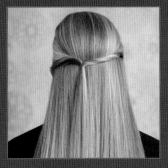

EASY TWISTED PULLBACK
47

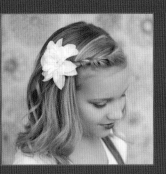

TWISTED BANGS OR FRINGE
49

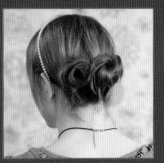

BOHO BUNS
53

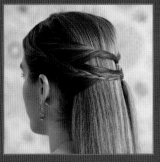

SIMPLE PULLBACKS & BRAID
57

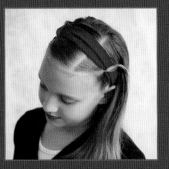

LINKED PONIES & SCARF
61

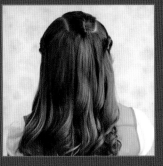

TRIPLE TWISTS
65

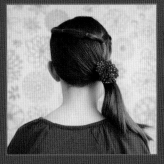

ELASTICS & PONYTAILS
69

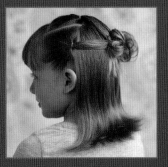

PONIES & MESSY BUN
73

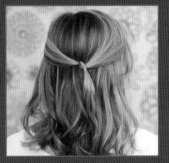

KNOT A HARD STYLE
77

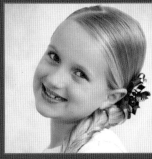

CHEVRON PONYTAIL
81

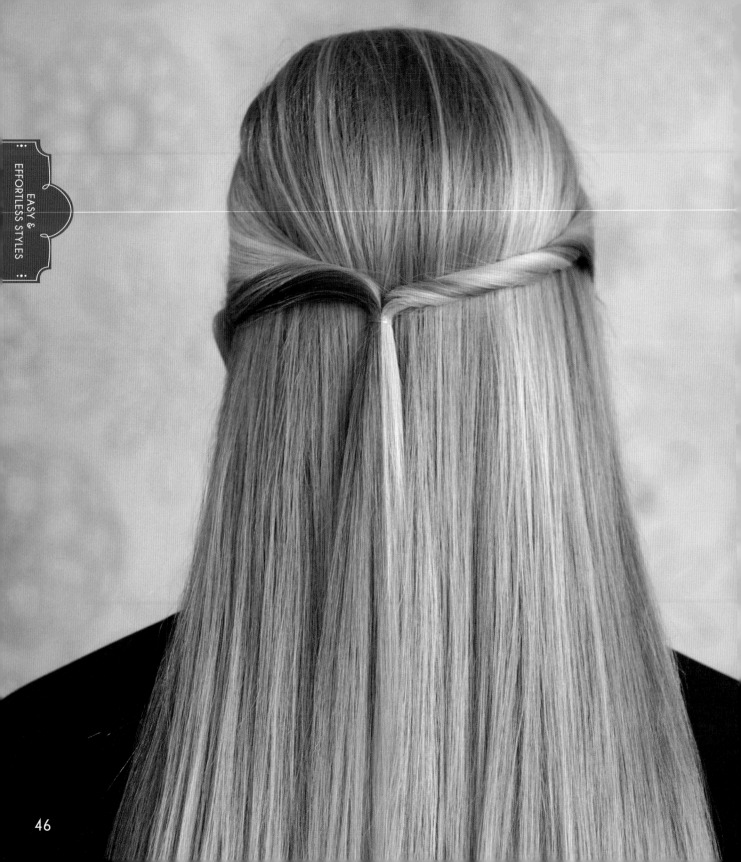

EASY TWISTED PULLBACK

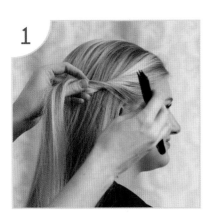

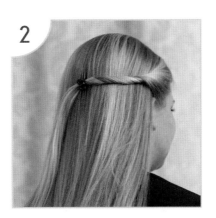

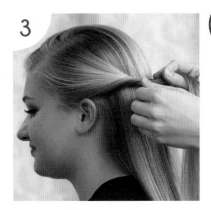

STEP 1 Make a part on the left side of the head. On the right side, gather the hair along the face line and near the ear. Begin twisting the hair inward toward the head.

STEP 2 Draw the hair back around to the middle of the head. Twist the section of hair as tight as desired and temporarily secure to the back of the head with a clip so it doesn't untwist.

STEP 3 On the left side, gather the hair along the hairline and ear and draw it back toward the other twist. Gently twist this section inward 2–3 times toward the head. You don't want this side as tightly twisted as the right side.

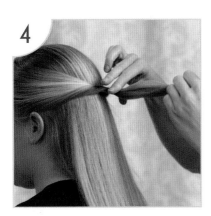

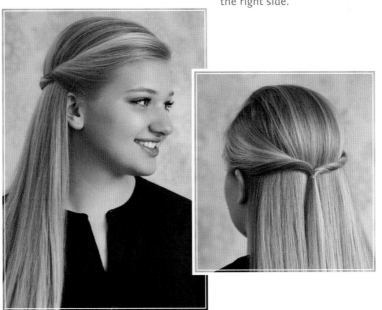

STEP 4 Remove the clip from step 2 and carefully join the twists together in back. Secure with a hair elastic. Mist entire hairstyle with hair spray.

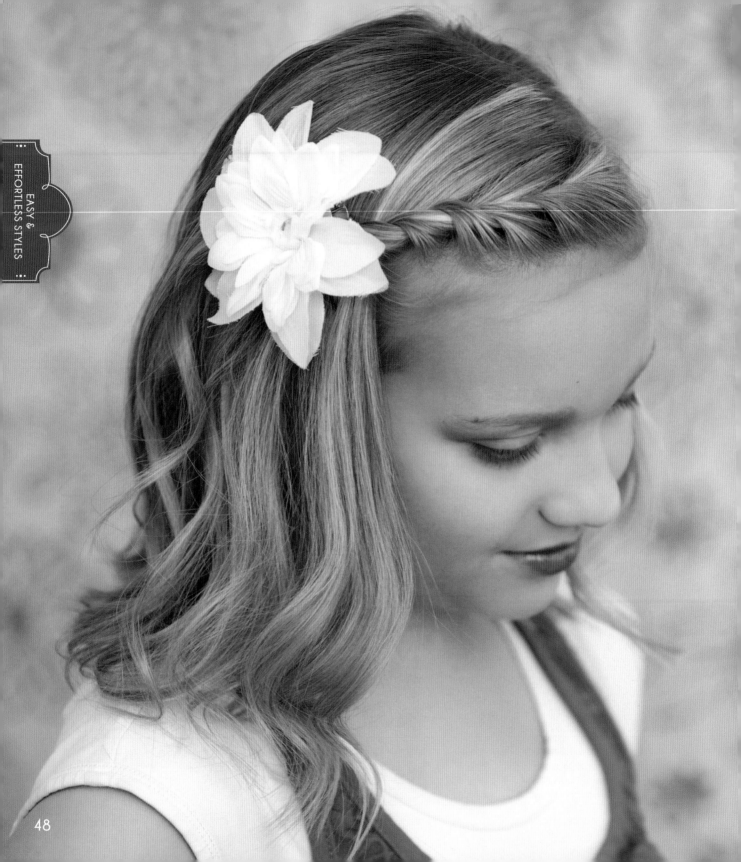

TWISTED BANGS OR FRINGE

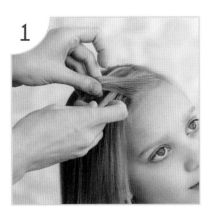

STEP 1 Make a part on the top of the head. Grasp a small section of hair along the front of the face and divide it into two sections. Cross the front section over the back section making an X.

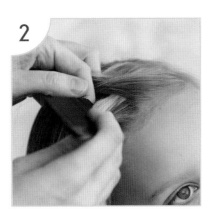

STEP 2 With the piece that is now in front or on the right, drop it so it joins the rest of the hair. With a comb or your fingers, grab that piece along with a small amount of hair from below.

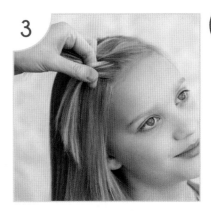

STEP 3 Draw all that hair upward so it crosses over the back piece, creating an X. They should then trade places and the back piece becomes the hair in front.

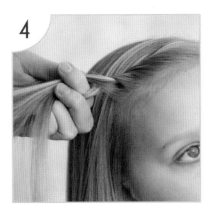

STEP 4 Continue the process of dropping the front piece, so you can incorporate more hair into that section, and twisting it over.

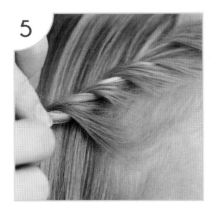

STEP 5 Add as much or as little hair to the twist as you like. This can continue clear around the head if you want.

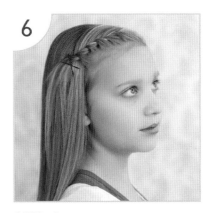

STEP 6 Secure the end of the twist with bobby pins. Use two and make an X for a more secure hold.

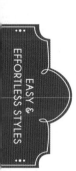

7

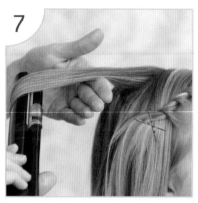

8

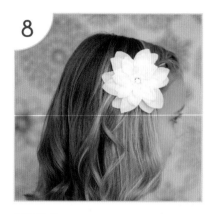

STEP 7 With a curling iron or flat iron, add some curl or waves to the remaining hair. Don't forget to use a heat-protecting serum before curling.

STEP 8 For an extra pretty look, add a flower or other accessory to hide the bobby pins. Mist entire hairstyle with hair spray.

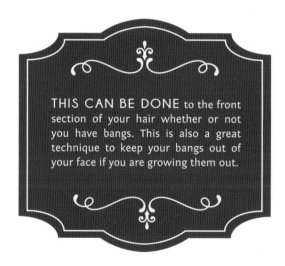

THIS CAN BE DONE to the front section of your hair whether or not you have bangs. This is also a great technique to keep your bangs out of your face if you are growing them out.

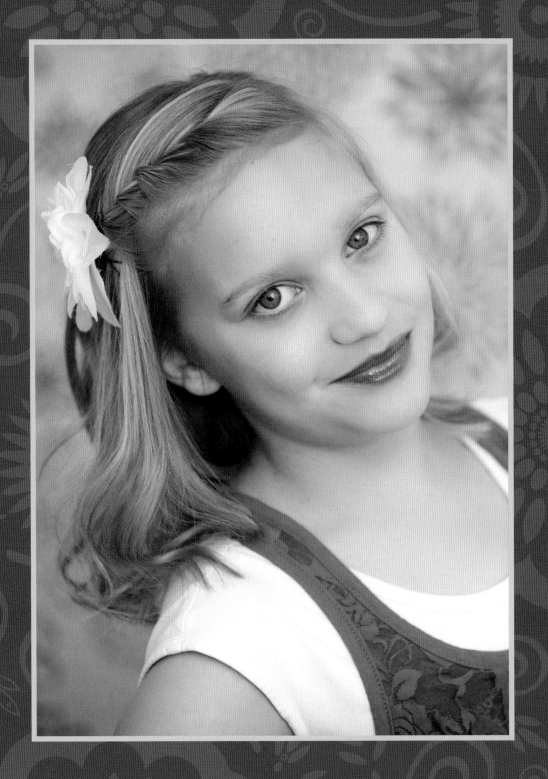

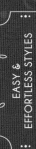

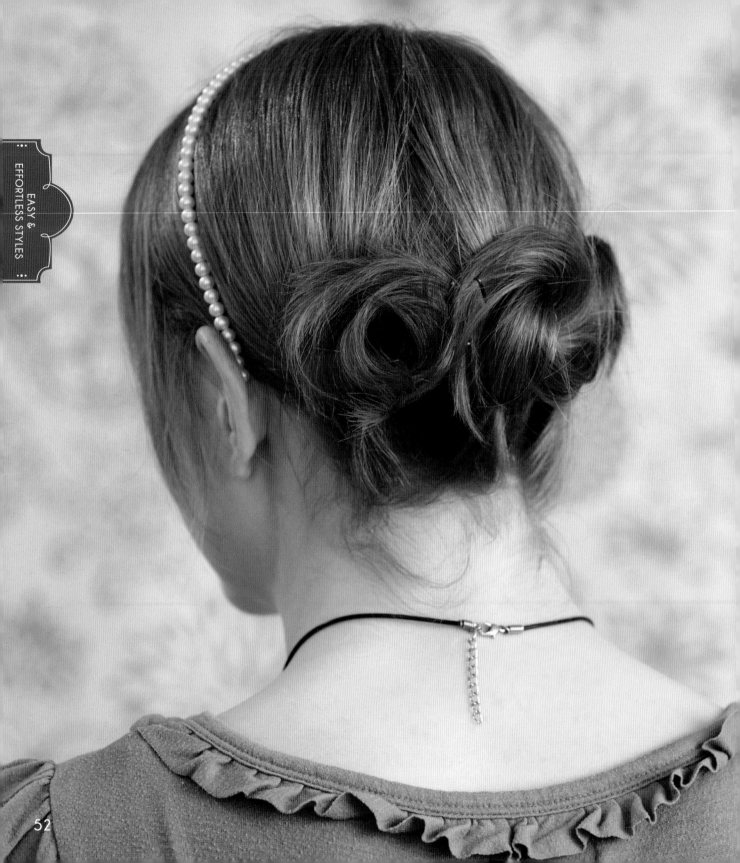

BOHO BUNS

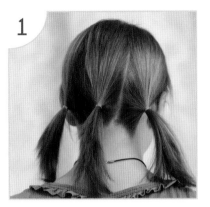

STEP 1 Divide the hair into three even sections and secure each one with a hair elastic in low ponytails at the nape of the neck.

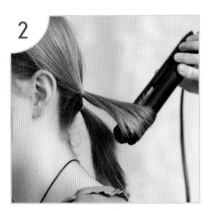

STEP 2 Starting with the left ponytail, curl the ends with a flat iron or curling iron.

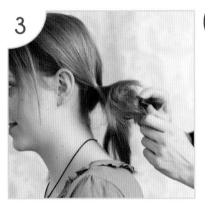

STEP 3 On the left, backcomb the ponytail a bit to add some volume. Then gently comb through the top layer of the ponytail to smooth it out.

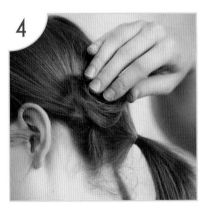

STEP 4 Wrap the hair in a clockwise direction to make a tiny bun or rosette to cover the elastic.

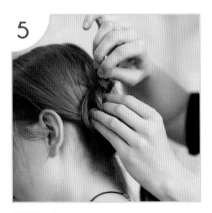

STEP 5 Secure the wrapped hair with bobby pins as needed. Let the ends spray out for a messier look.

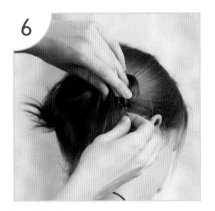

STEP 6 Repeat steps 2–5 on the middle and right ponytails creating two more rosettes. Secure as needed with bobby pins.

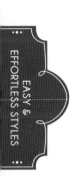

7

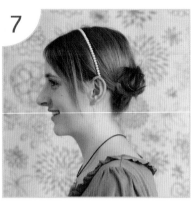

STEP 7 To dress up the style, add a headband or scarf. Mist entire hairstyle with hair spray.

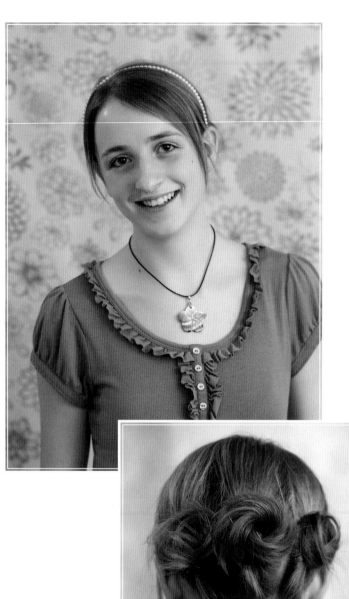

ALTHOUGH THIS STYLE can be done with longer hair, this style works best on shorter hair to achieve a messier and carefree look. If you wish to dress it up a bit more add a pretty headband.

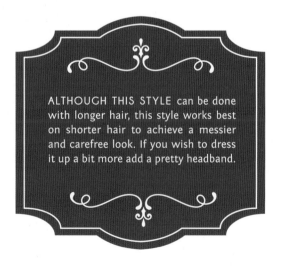

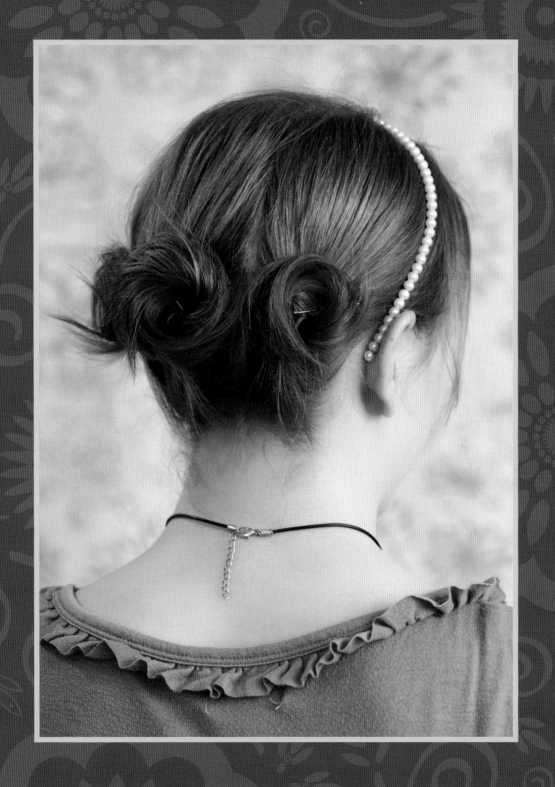

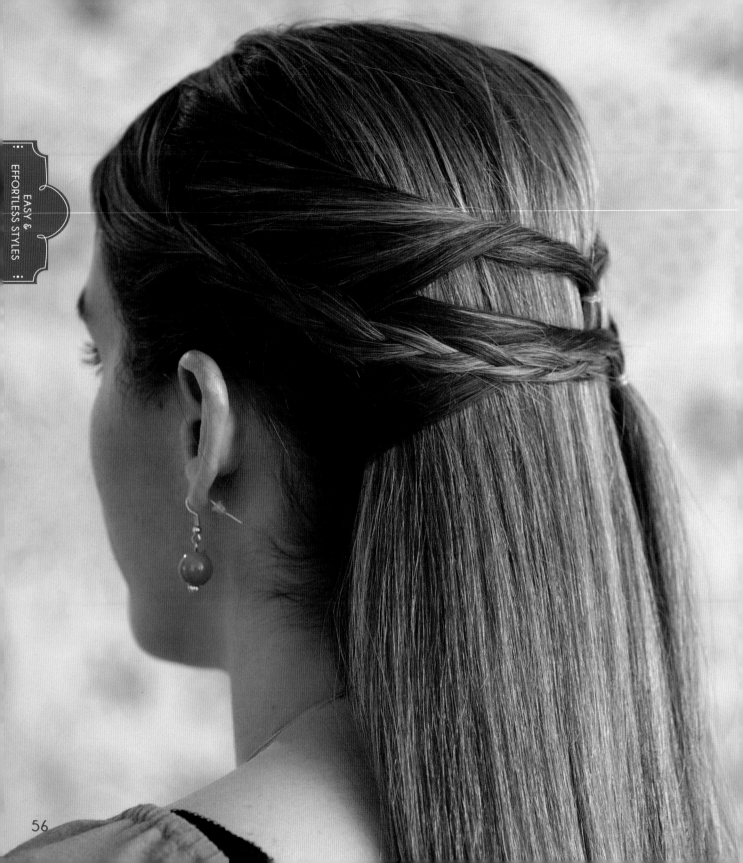

SIMPLE PULLBACKS & BRAID

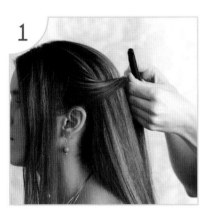

STEP 1 Make an off-center part on the right side of the head. On the left side of the head, section out hair in front of the ear at the hairline. Draw it back toward the right side of the head. Leave the hair above it at the temple hanging freely for now.

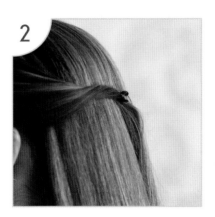

STEP 2 Slightly twist the section of hair inward, and with a small claw clip, secure it to the back of the head.

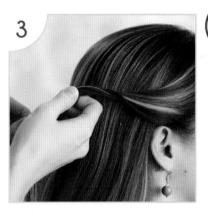

STEP 3 On the right side, section out hair along the face and the right ear and draw it backward. Slightly twist this section of hair.

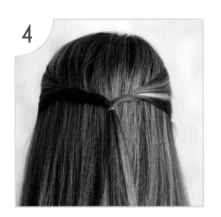

STEP 4 Remove the clip holding the left section of hair, and join the two sections. Secure them with an elastic, so that it sits slightly to the right side of the head.

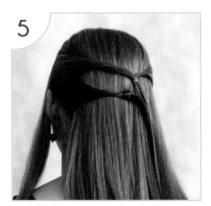

STEP 5 Section out a small amount of hair from behind the left ear below the section from step 1. Temporarily secure it in back with a small claw clip.

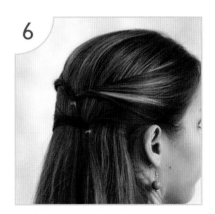

STEP 6 Section out a small amount of hair on the right side behind the ear. Slightly twist it and join it with the section from the left. Secure the two pieces together with an elastic so that the elastic sits further right than the first elastic.

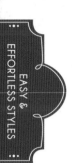

7

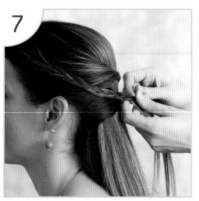

8

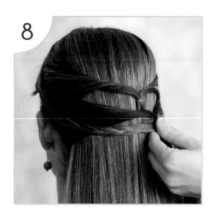

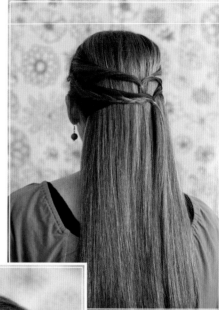

STEP 7 With the remaining hair by the left temple, make a regular 3-strand braid as shown on page 22.

STEP 8 Braid the hair until it will reach back to the bottom elastic from step 6. Don't pull the braid tight or straight back. Loosely drape it back over the bottom section of hair. Secure the braid with another elastic to the elastic in step 6. Mist entire hairstyle with hair spray.

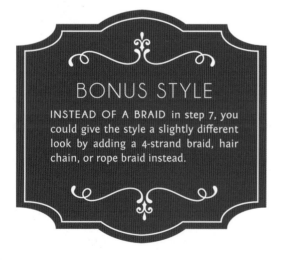

BONUS STYLE

INSTEAD OF A BRAID in step 7, you could give the style a slightly different look by adding a 4-strand braid, hair chain, or rope braid instead.

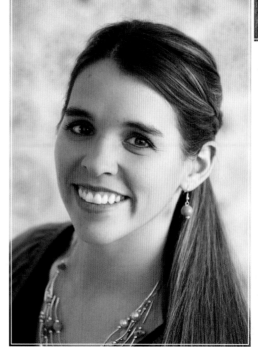

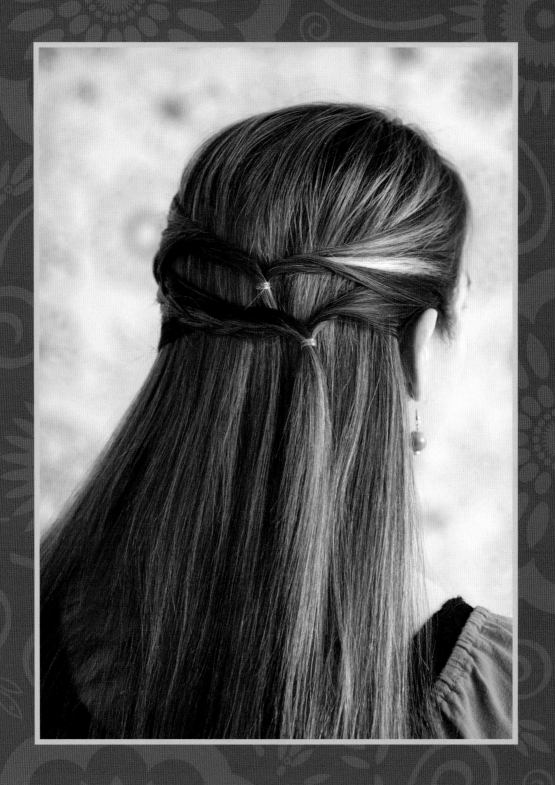

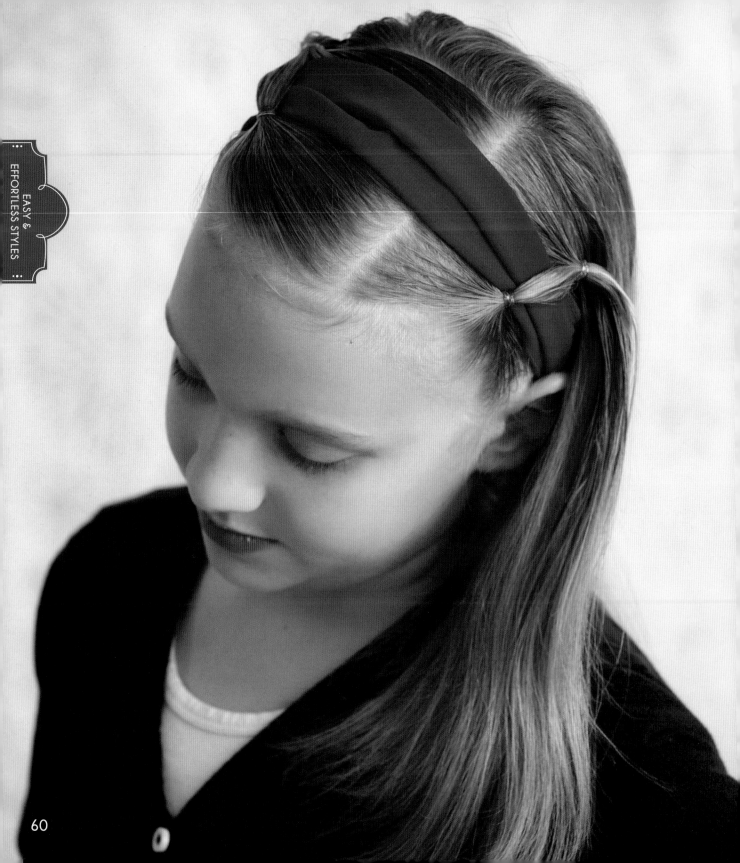

LINKED PONIES & SCARF

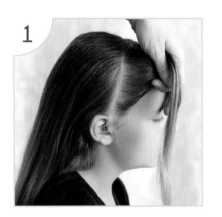

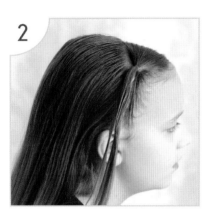

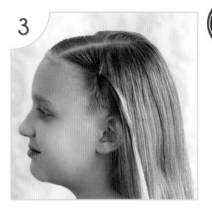

STEP 1 On the top of the head, make an off-center part on the left. Branching off that, part down to the right ear.

STEP 2 With that section, make a small ponytail that sits near the hairline. Secure with an elastic close to the scalp.

STEP 3 On the left side of the head, make a part down to the ear. Make another ponytail, securing it close to the scalp so it is also positioned near the hairline.

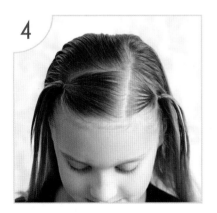

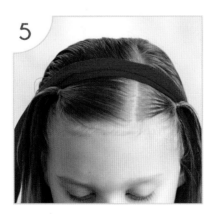

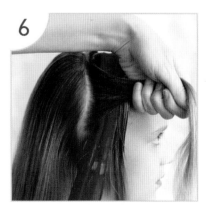

STEP 4 The ponytails should sit about even on each side of the head, back from the temples.

STEP 5 Place a scarf, wide ribbon, or headband just behind the ponytails. It should cover up the part that runs ear to ear.

STEP 6 On the right side, just behind the scarf, part out another section of hair.

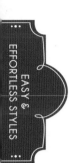

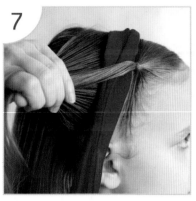

STEP 7 Smooth out the hair behind the scarf and take hold of the ponytail in front of the scarf.

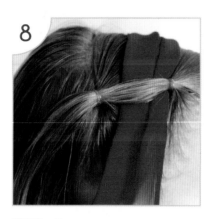

STEP 8 Join these two sections together and secure with an elastic, making a new ponytail. Be sure the elastic is wrapped tightly and sits close to the scalp. Hair should now pass over the scarf.

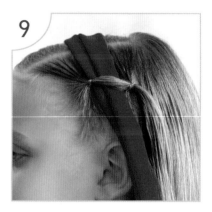

STEP 9 Repeat steps 6–8 on the left side of the head.

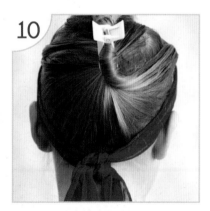

STEP 10 Twist the hair in back up and out of the way and temporarily secure with a clip. Tie the scarf in a knot at the nape of the neck. Remove the clip and let the hair down to cover the knot. If desired add a little or a lot of curl to the hair down in back. Mist entire hairstyle with hair spray.

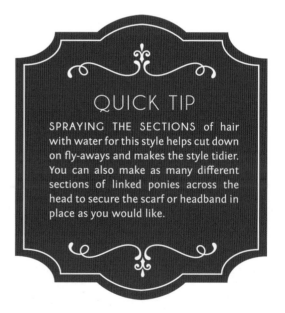

QUICK TIP

SPRAYING THE SECTIONS of hair with water for this style helps cut down on fly-aways and makes the style tidier. You can also make as many different sections of linked ponies across the head to secure the scarf or headband in place as you would like.

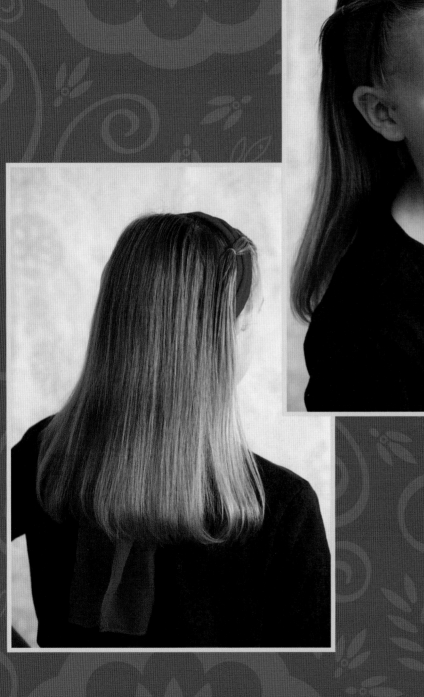

63

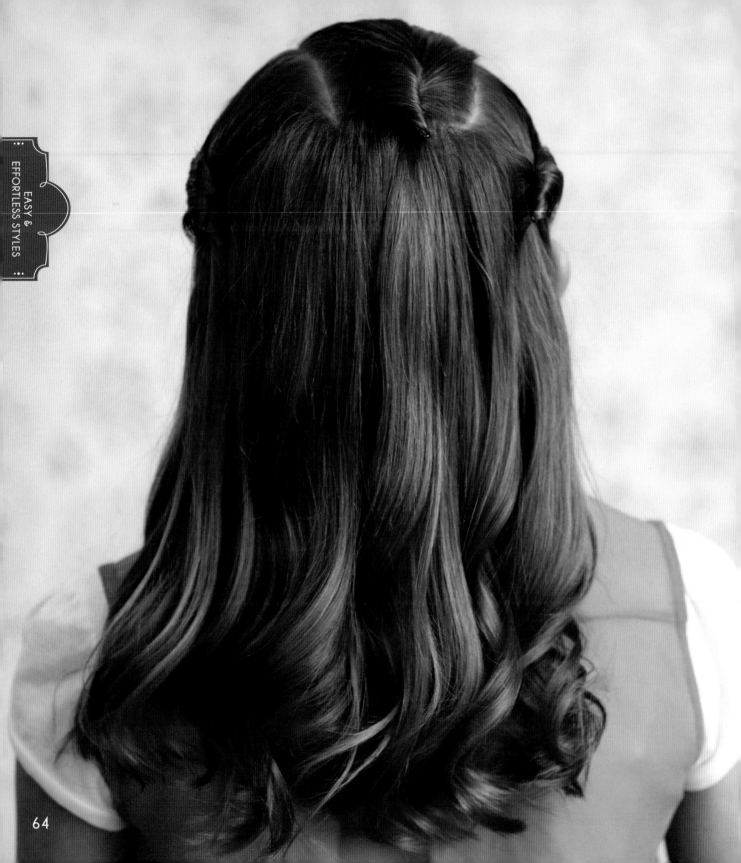

TRIPLE TWISTS

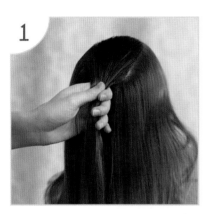

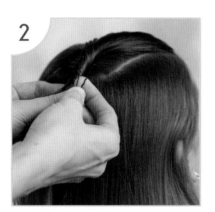

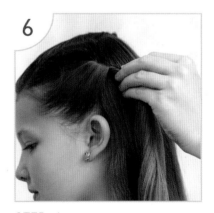

STEP 1 On the very top of the head, section off a rectangle of hair. Start the parts from about the inner edge of the eyebrow straight back to the crown.

STEP 2 Tightly twist the section of hair to the right. Take a bobby pin and open the end up wide.

STEP 3 Place the open ends of the bobby pin over the twist, so the ends straddle the twist. Push the bobby pin in toward the front of the face for a firm hold.

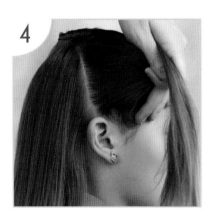

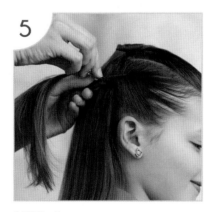

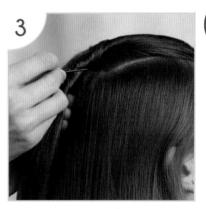

STEP 4 On the right side of the head, make a part from the crown down to the right ear.

STEP 5 Twist the hair in toward the head and secure with a bobby pin as directed in step 3.

STEP 6 Repeat on the left side of the head and secure the twist with a bobby pin.

7

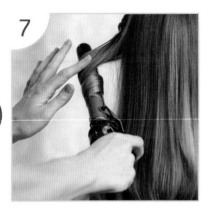

STEP 7 To dress the style up, curl the hair that is down in back. Mist entire hairstyle with hair spray.

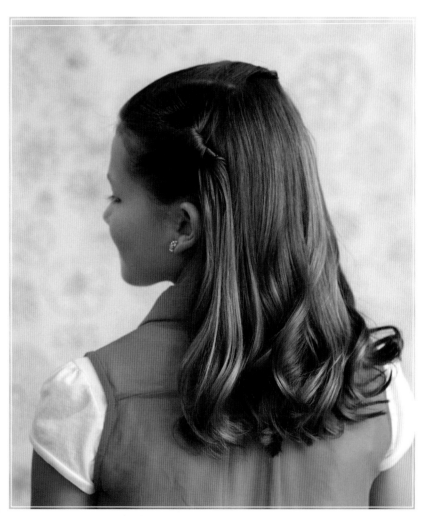

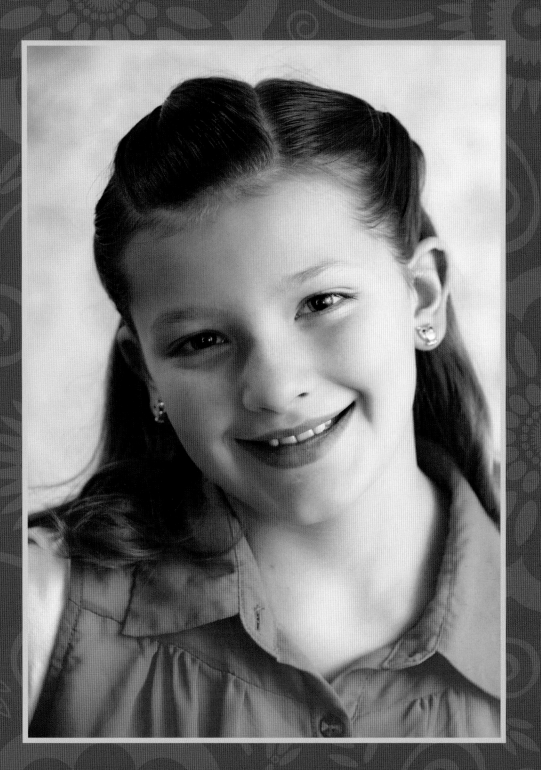

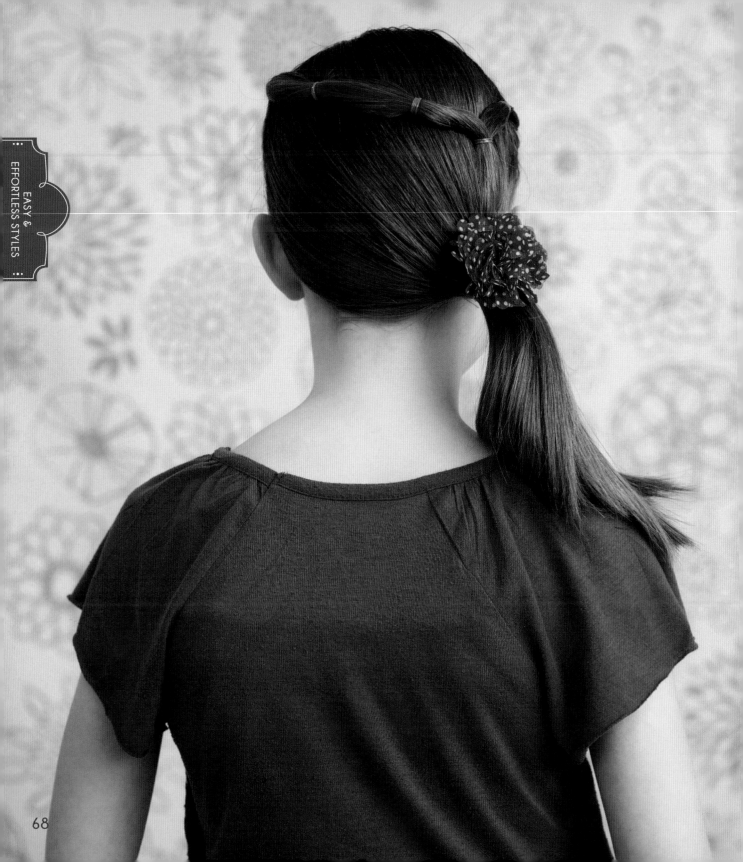

ELASTICS & PONYTAILS

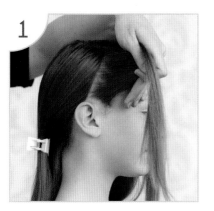

STEP 1 Make a part on the top right side of the head back to the crown. Make another part branching off it down to the front of the right ear.

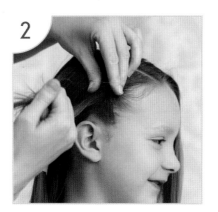

STEP 2 Gather this section of hair into a ponytail and secure with a colored hair elastic.

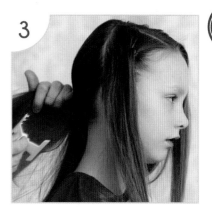

STEP 3 Right behind the first ponytail, part out another section of hair from the crown down to the back of the right ear and with a clip hold the rest of the hair out of the way.

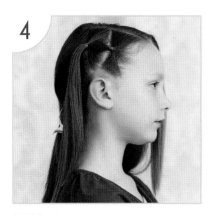

STEP 4 Gather this new section of hair into a second ponytail, incorporating the ponytail from step 2. Secure it with another colored hair elastic.

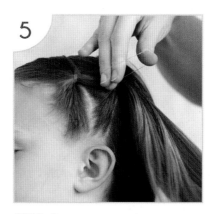

STEP 5 Repeat steps 2–4 on the left side of the head, making two little ponytails. Be sure the parts running down to the left ear are a continuation of the ones on the right side of the head.

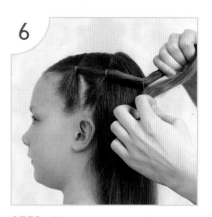

STEP 6 About two inches behind the second elastic on the left side of the head, add a third elastic. Do not add any hair. Simply wrap a colored elastic around the hair about the same distance apart as the front ponytails.

69

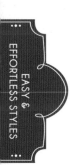

7

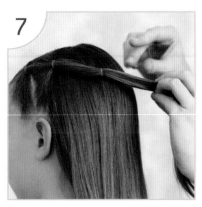

STEP 7 Add another colored elastic a few inches behind the one in step 6. Again, do not add any hair. Just wrap the elastic around the hair. You should now have four colored elastics along the left side.

8

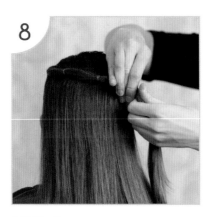

STEP 8 Next, take the ponytail from the left and the ponytail from the right and join them together on the right side of the head. Secure with another colored elastic.

9

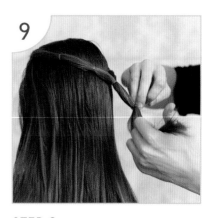

STEP 9 A few inches below the elastic in step 8, without adding any hair, wrap another colored elastic around the ponytail shaft.

10

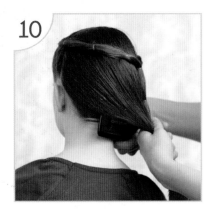

STEP 10 Gather the remaining hair into a low ponytail behind the right ear and secure with an elastic. Add a flower or accessory to cover the elastic. Mist entire hairstyle with hair spray.

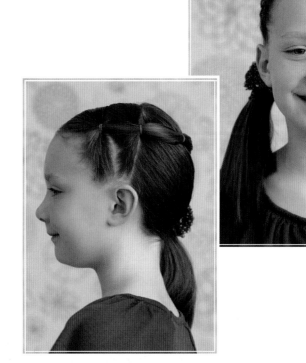

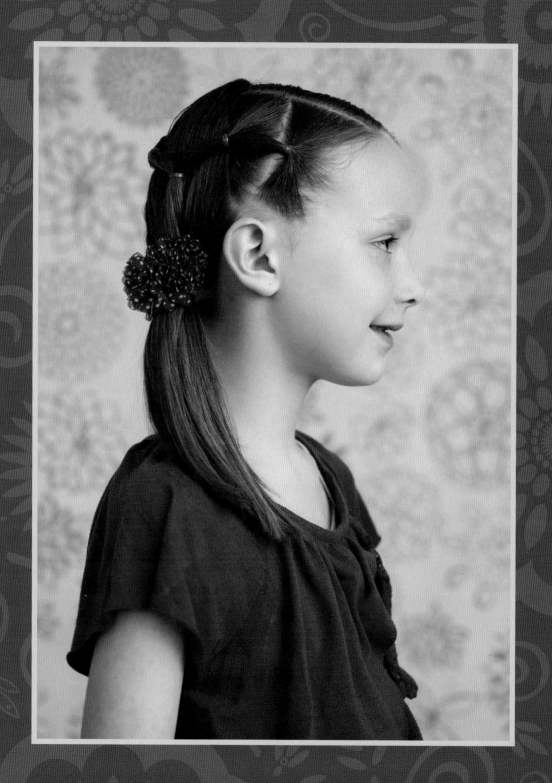

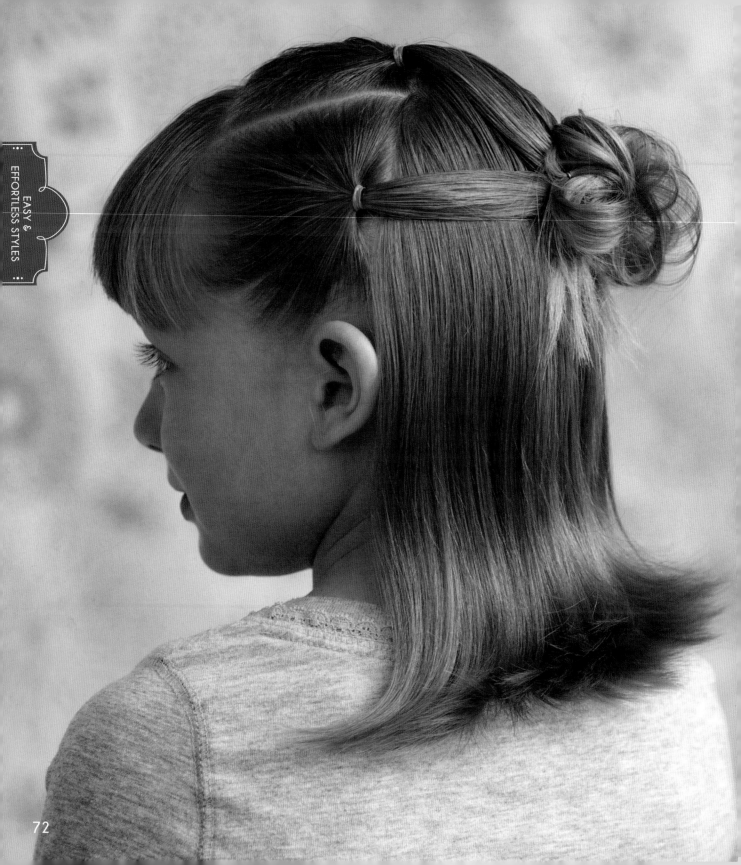

PONIES & MESSY BUN

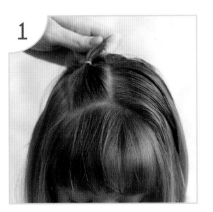

STEP 1 Part the hair down the middle of the head back to the crown. Make a part parallel to it about two inches to the right and then along the crown. Gather that rectangular section of hair into a small ponytail and secure with an elastic.

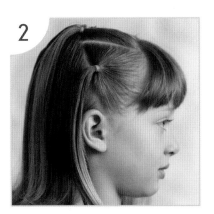

STEP 2 With the remaining hair on the right, part down to the ear and make another small ponytail. Secure the ponytail with another elastic.

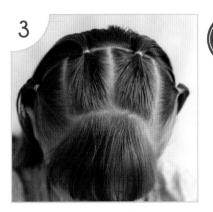

STEP 3 Repeat the above steps on the left side of the head. You will end up with four small ponytails along the crown.

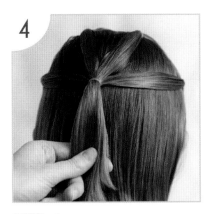

STEP 4 Bring the ends of all four ponytails to the center back of the head. Secure them all together in one ponytail with another elastic.

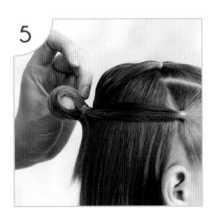

STEP 5 Wrap a second elastic around the base of the ponytail in back. Once the elastic is fairly tight, don't pull the ponytail all the way through the last time. The ponytail will form a small loop.

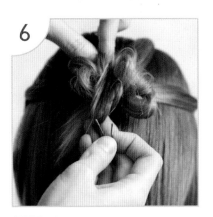

STEP 6 As shown on page 38, pull the loop apart to create a small messy bun. Use small bobby pins to secure the messy bun. Arrange the bun and the "tails" that spray out from below it as desired. Add curl to the remaining hair in back if you like.

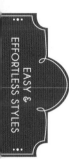

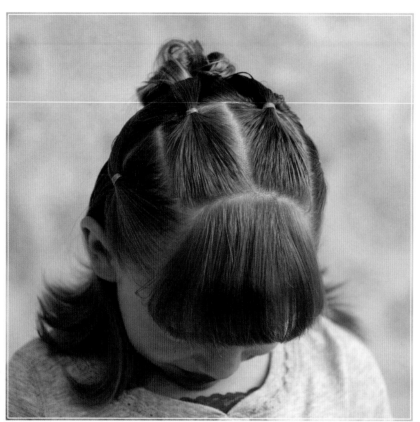

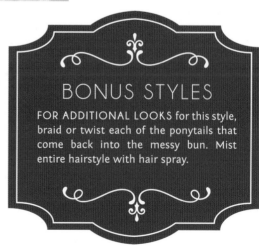

BONUS STYLES

FOR ADDITIONAL LOOKS for this style, braid or twist each of the ponytails that come back into the messy bun. Mist entire hairstyle with hair spray.

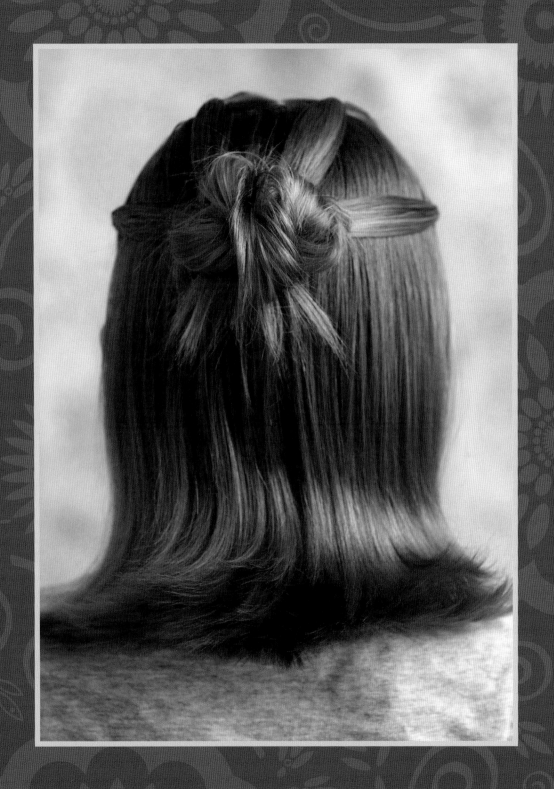

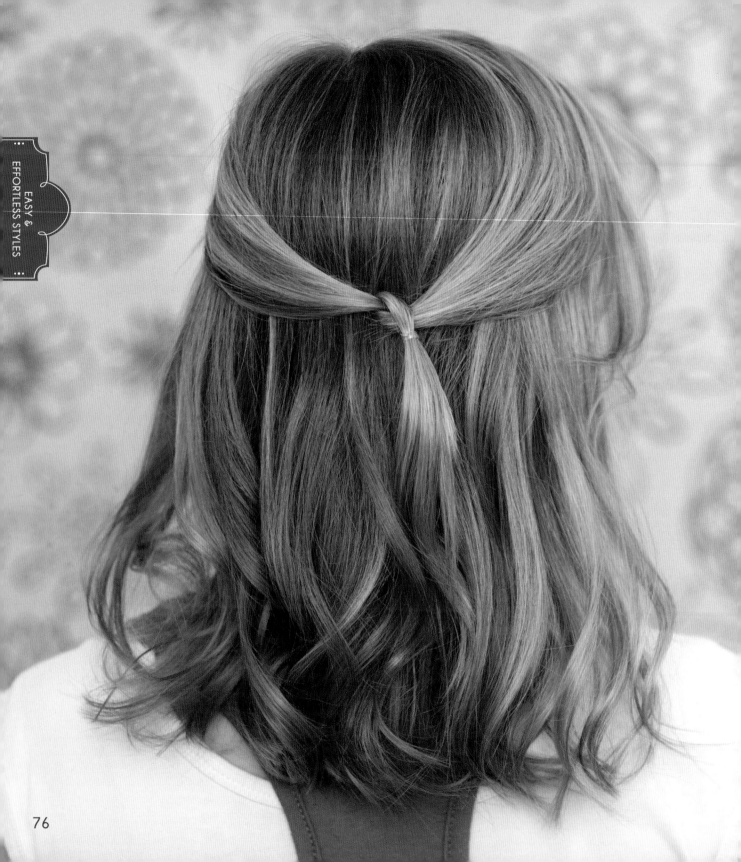

KNOT A HARD STYLE

1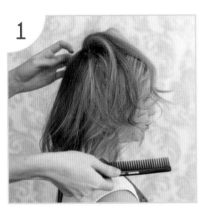

STEP 1 Back comb several small sections of hair at the crown for extra volume.

2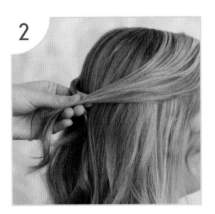

STEP 2 Take a small section of hair along the left temple and from the right side of the head and draw them backward. If you have bangs, you can leave them out and style them as you normally do.

3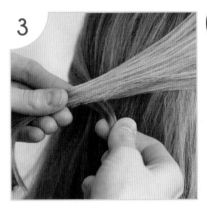

STEP 3 Cross the right piece of hair over the left piece to form an X.

4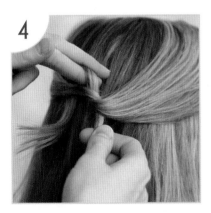

STEP 4 Pass the right piece under the left piece of hair and draw it upward.

5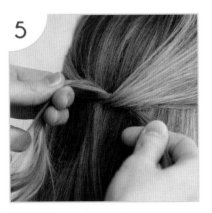

STEP 5 Pull gently on each piece to tighten the hair.

6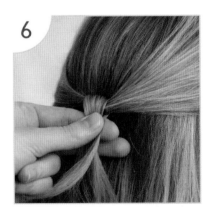

STEP 6 Take the left piece of hair and lay it on top of the right piece.

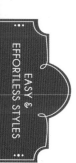

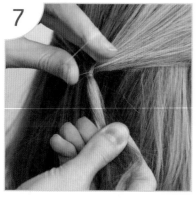

STEP 7 With a clear elastic, secure them together to form a small knot.

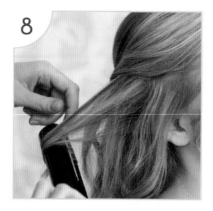

STEP 8 For a bit of added texture, add some curl to the remaining hair and bangs. Mist entire hairstyle with hair spray.

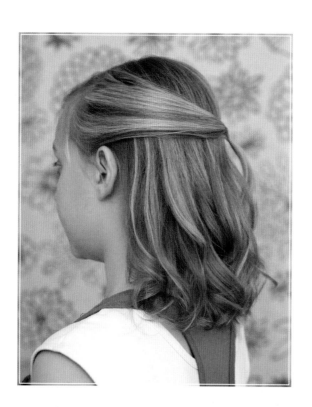

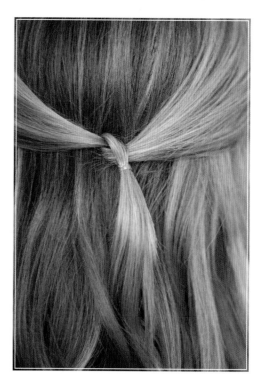

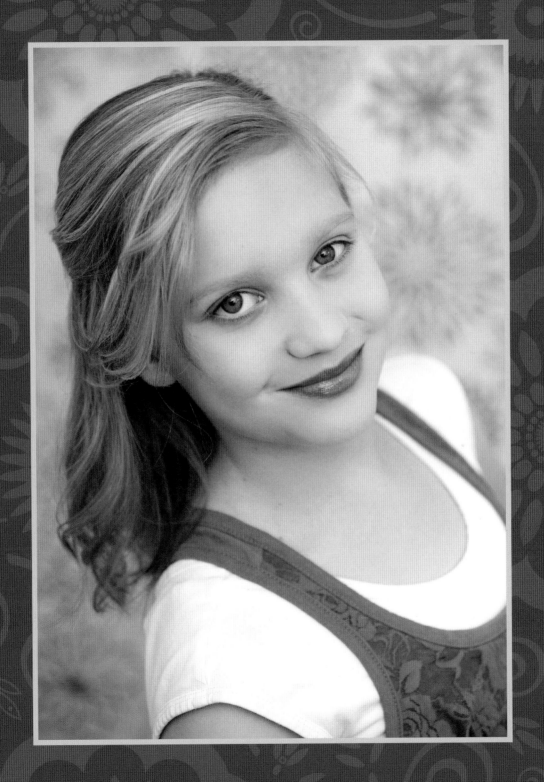

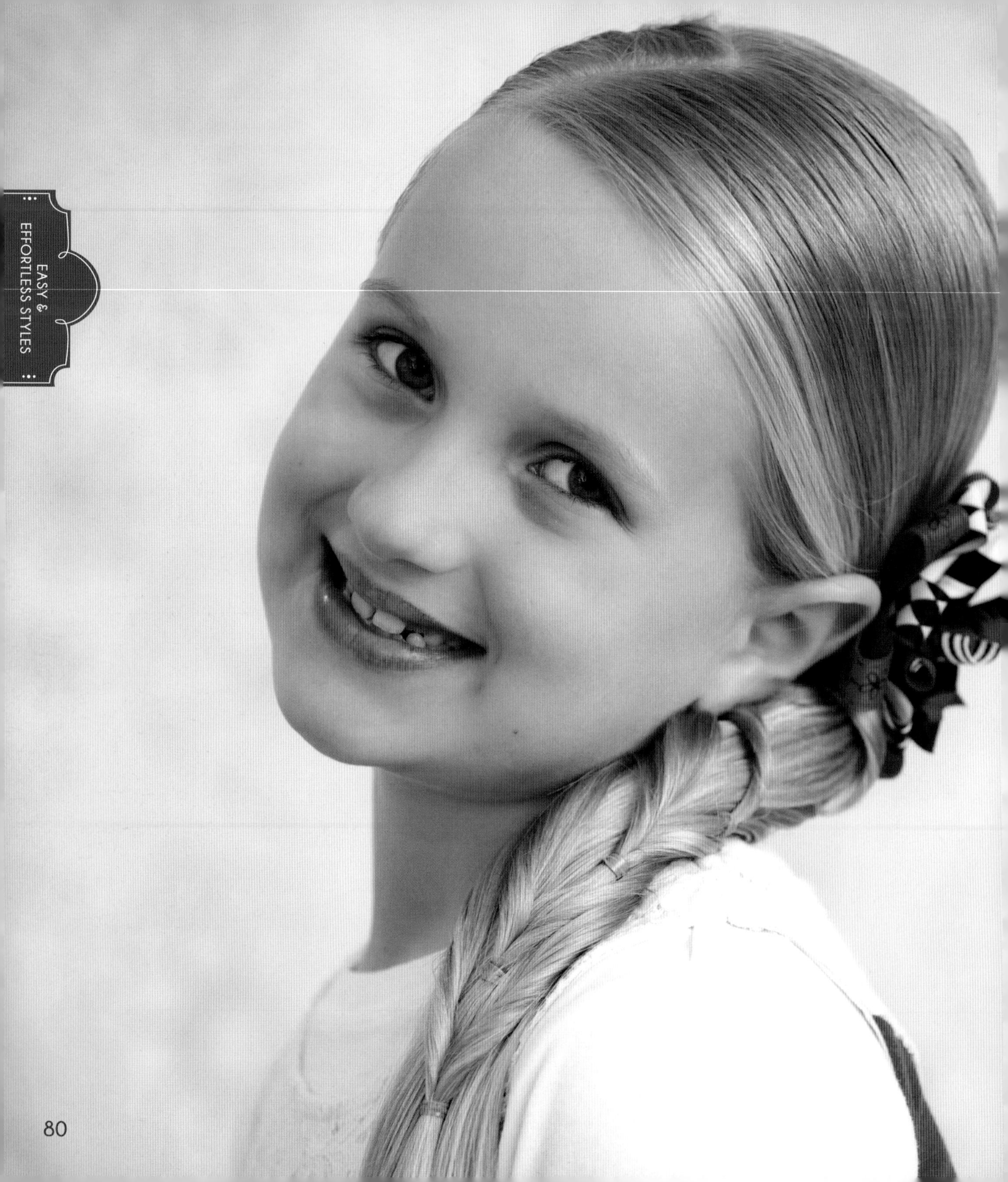

CHEVRON PONYTAIL

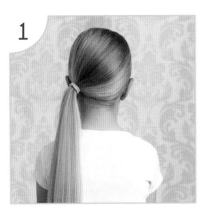

STEP 1 Gather all the hair and make a ponytail behind the left ear.

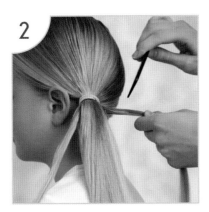

STEP 2 From each side of the ponytail, section out a piece of hair. Mist them with water or hair spray to reduce fly-aways.

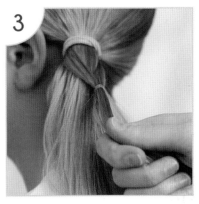

STEP 3 Bring the two pieces of hair over the top of the ponytail. Pinch them together and secure them with a colored hair elastic so it forms a V on top of the ponytail.

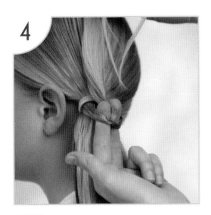

STEP 4 Flip the ponytail by putting your fingers underneath the colored elastic and up through the middle of the V.

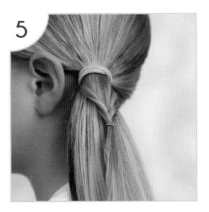

STEP 5 Pull the ends of the small ponytail through the "hole" with your fingers and it will give the two small pieces a twisted look.

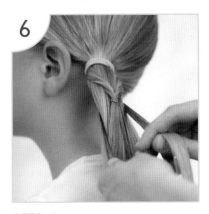

STEP 6 Repeat the process, sectioning out two small pieces of hair from each side of the big ponytail.

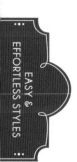

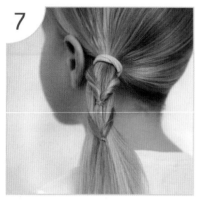

STEP 7 Join the pieces together with another colored elastic.

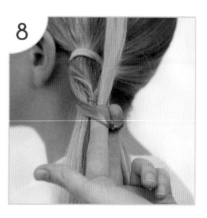

STEP 8 Flip the ponytail through again so the strands become twisted.

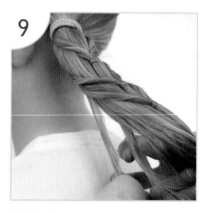

STEP 9 Continue steps 2–5 as many times as desired, working your way down the ponytail. As you get further down the ponytail, it might help to cross the small sections of hair underneath the ponytail first before joining them in front. It seems to help the mini-ponytails lay a bit better on top.

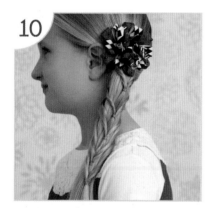

STEP 10 Add a fun hair accessory to cover the base of the ponytail. Or if you prefer, before starting step 2, wrap the base of the ponytail with hair as shown on page 36. Mist entire hairstyle with hair spray.

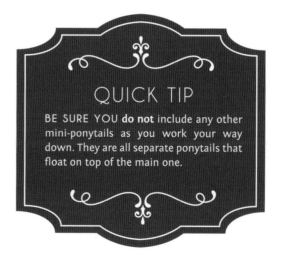

QUICK TIP

BE SURE YOU **do not** include any other mini-ponytails as you work your way down. They are all separate ponytails that float on top of the main one.

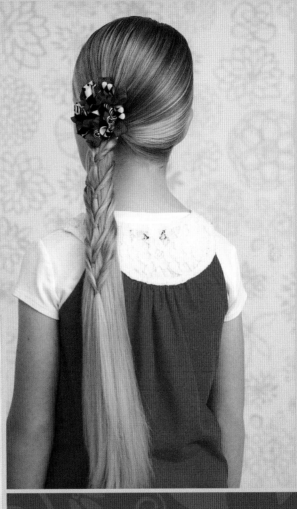

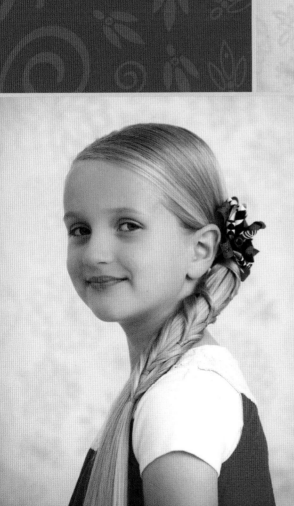

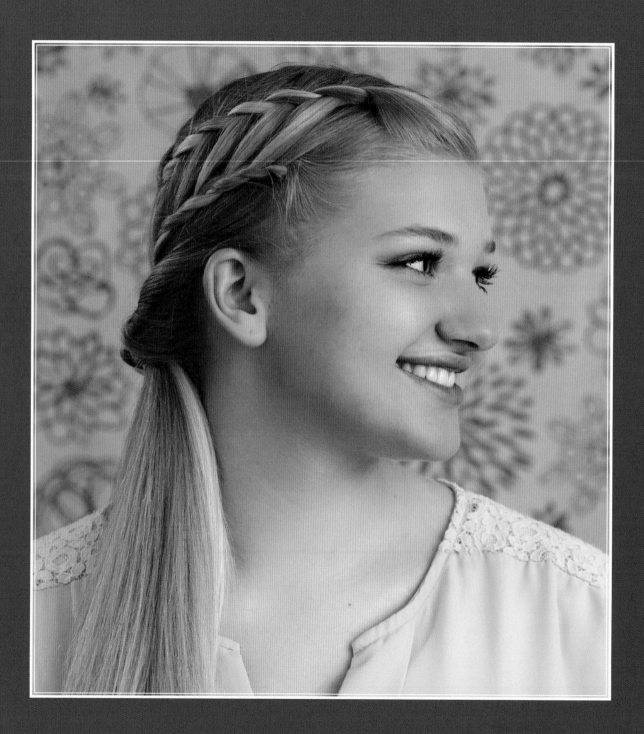

CHAPTER 4

Everyday & Any Occasion Styles

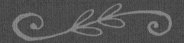

Everyday & Any Occasion Styles

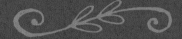

These styles are a little more advanced and combine more techniques. Some may require more time and effort than others.

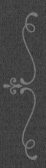

THE STYLES in this section are perfect for school, work, or just about any occasion. They combine more of the basic techniques taught in Chapter 2. Depending on your skill level, they may take a little longer than the styles from the previous chapter. These styles are meant to inspire and give you confidence in creating more involved hairstyles. Feel free to follow them exactly, or put your own spin on them. Have fun trying new things. I believe as long as you like how it turns out, that's what is important. Also remember, we tend to be our own worst critic. There have been times when I created a style that I really didn't like but got tons of compliments on it—so you never know! Just keep practicing and trying new things. The sky's the limit!

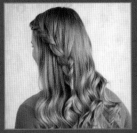

WAVES & PANCAKED LACE BRAID

89

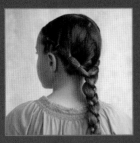

LINKED PONIES & UNEVEN BRAID

93

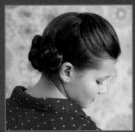

BEAUTIFUL BRAIDED BUNS

97

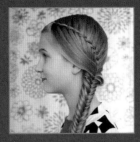

WATERFALL TWIST & FISHBONE

101

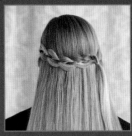

4-STRAND BRAID WRAP

105

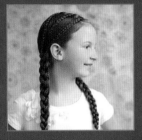

PRETTY POCAHONTAS BRAIDS

109

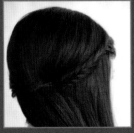

SIDESWEPT FISHBONE BRAID

113

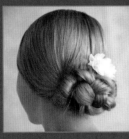

BRAIDED CHIGNON

117

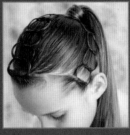

TRI-CHAIN PONYTAIL

121

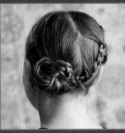

NESTED BRAIDS & BUN

125

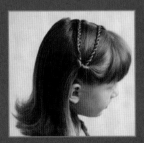

MINI BRAID & TWIST

129

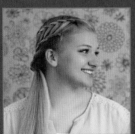

LADDER BRAID FLIPPED PONYTAIL

133

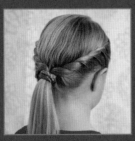

FRENCH ROPE TWISTS

137

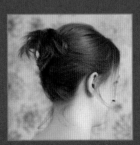

THE PEACOCK TWIST

141

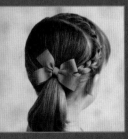

SIDE PONY & FRENCH BRAID

145

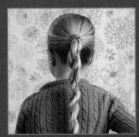

MICRO BRAIDS WITH A TWIST

147

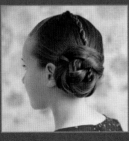

UNEVEN ROPE TWIST & BUN

151

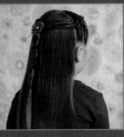

FAUX FISHBONES

155

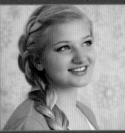

PANCAKED SIDESWEPT FRENCH BRAID

159

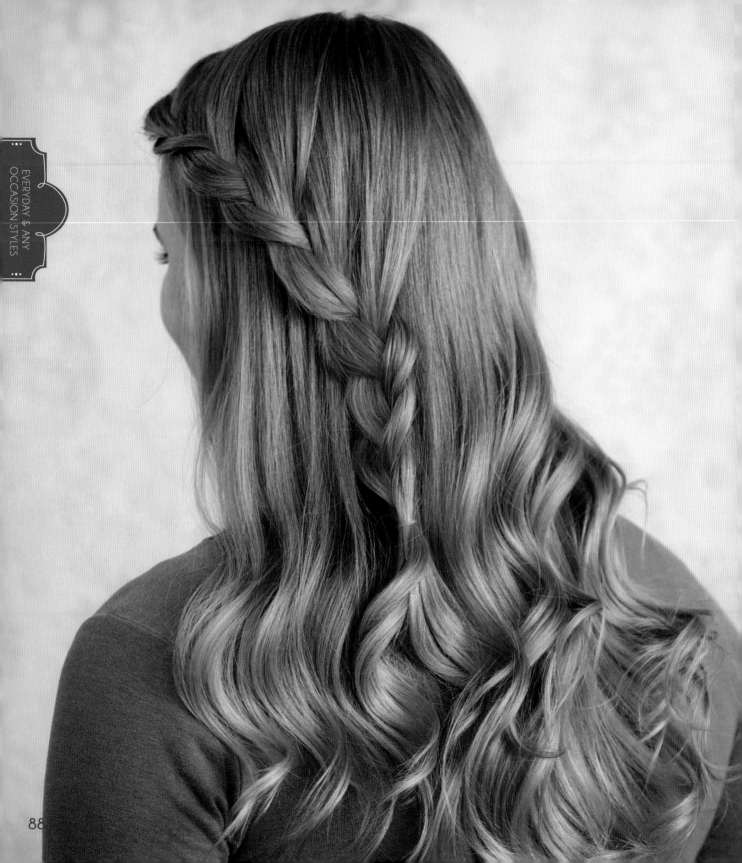

WAVES & PANCAKED LACE BRAID

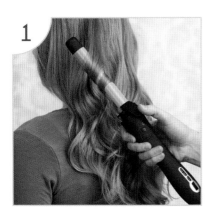

STEP 1 Begin by loosely curling the bottom half of all the hair to achieve a nice wave.

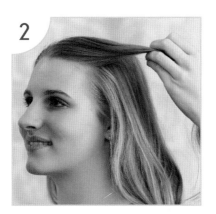

STEP 2 On the left side of the head take a section of hair above the forehead along the hairline and divide it into three pieces.

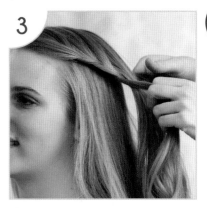

STEP 3 Loosely plait a lace braid as shown on page 26, but take bigger sections and use dry hair. Remember to only add hair to the top of the braid.

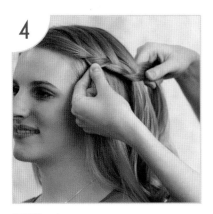

STEP 4 After braiding a few full rotations of the braid, gently tug on the bottom edges of the braid to give it a thicker appearance.

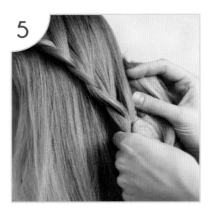

STEP 5 Once you've added 5–6 thick sections into the braid or have reached the crown, stop adding hair and continue braiding a regular 3-strand braid. Secure the end with a clear hair elastic.

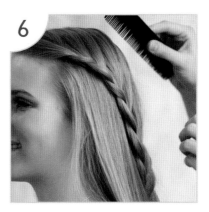

STEP 6 Smooth any bumps on top and pancake the braid further if you desire. Mist entire hairstyle with hair spray.

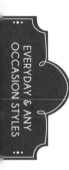

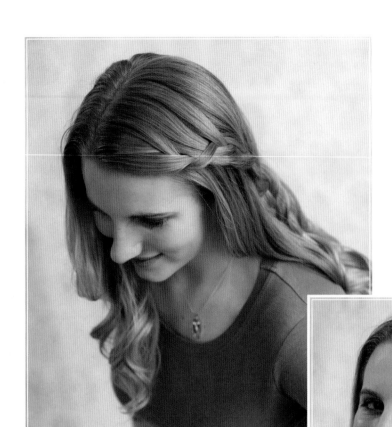

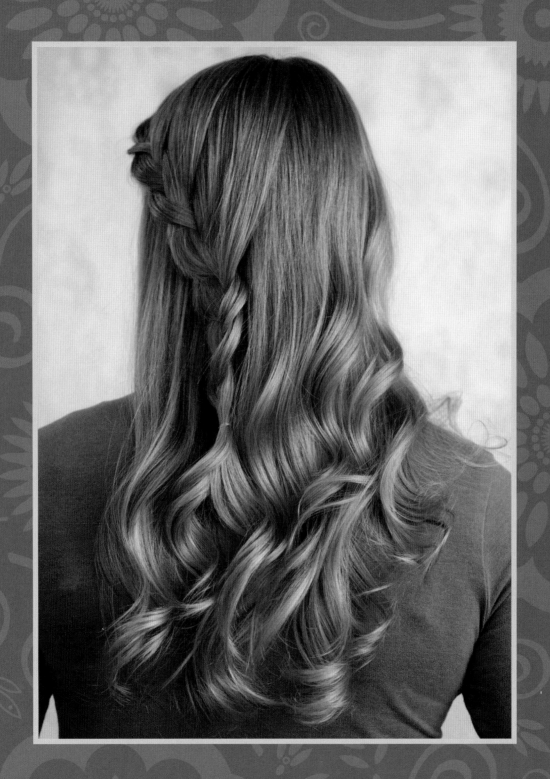

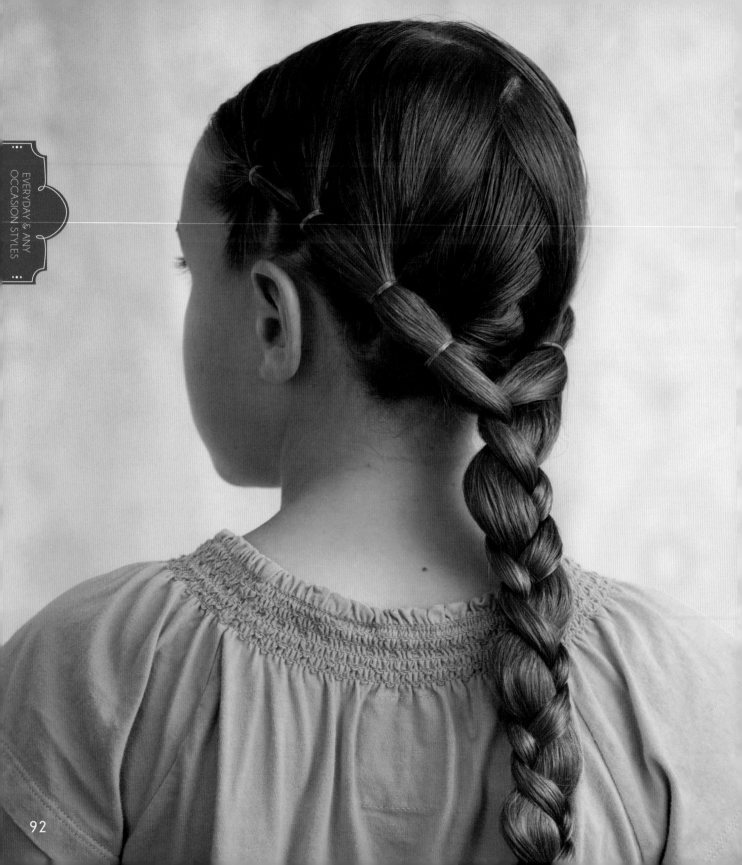

LINKED PONIES & UNEVEN BRAID

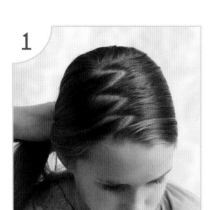

1

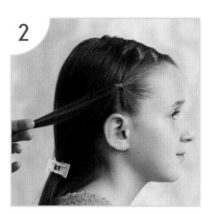

2

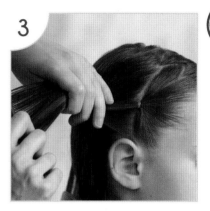

3

STEP 1 Using the end of a rat-tail comb, create a zigzag part down the middle of the head. Start at the forehead and continue back to the nape of the neck.

STEP 2 From the zigzag part down to the front of the right ear, make a part. Gather that hair into a small ponytail and secure with a colored hair elastic close to the scalp.

STEP 3 Make another part running from the top of the head down to just behind the right ear. Gather the hair from that section and include the ponytail from step 2. Secure all that hair with a colored hair elastic.

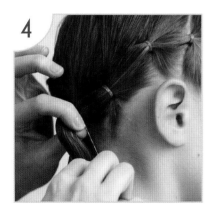

4

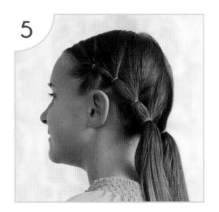

5

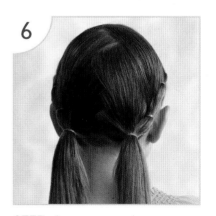

6

STEP 4 Repeat the process two more times, parting out hair and adding the ponytail from the section in front of it. The fourth elastic should be right at the base of the neck and there should be no more hair to add.

STEP 5 Repeat the above steps on the left side of the head. Try to make the parts even with the ones from the right side. You will have four connected ponytails on the left side when you are done.

STEP 6 You can be done with the style if you wish and wrap the base of the ponytails with hair (see page 36), or add some cute accessories to cover the elastics.

7

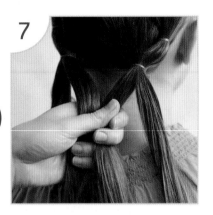

8

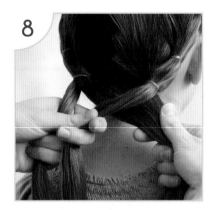

9

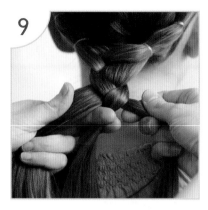

STEP 7 Divide a small section of hair out of the left side of the left ponytail. And do the same on the right ponytail. Bring the two inner sections of the ponytails together to create one section. You will be creating an uneven 3-strand braid (see page 25).

STEP 8 Begin braiding by drawing the outer right strand over the two middle sections (that act as one section now.)

STEP 9 As you proceed to braid be sure to pull the first several sections tight so the braid cinches right up to the hairline.

10

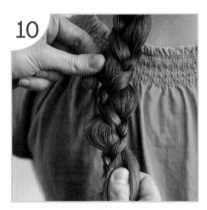

STEP 10 Continue the uneven 3-strand braid down as far as you can. While holding the tip of the braid with one hand, gently start pulling on the thicker sections of the braid with the other. Secure the braid with an elastic once desired look is achieved. Mist entire hairstyle with hair spray.

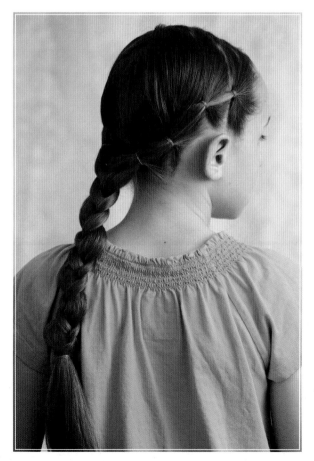

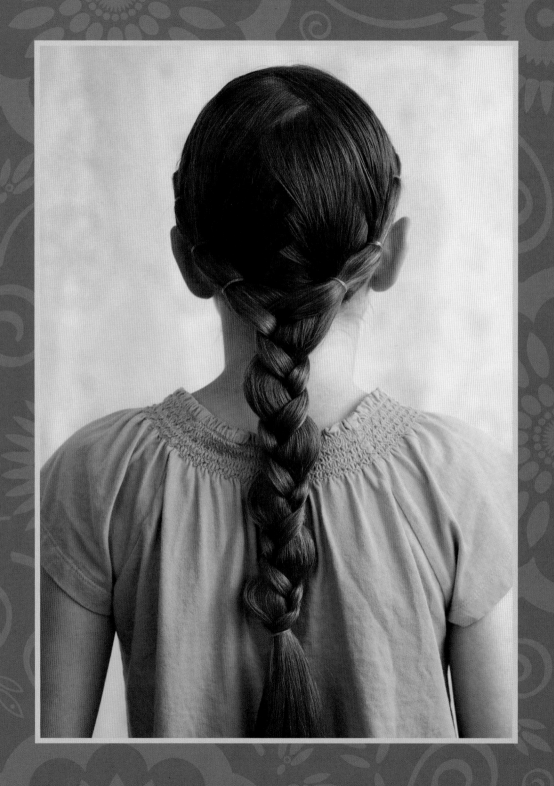

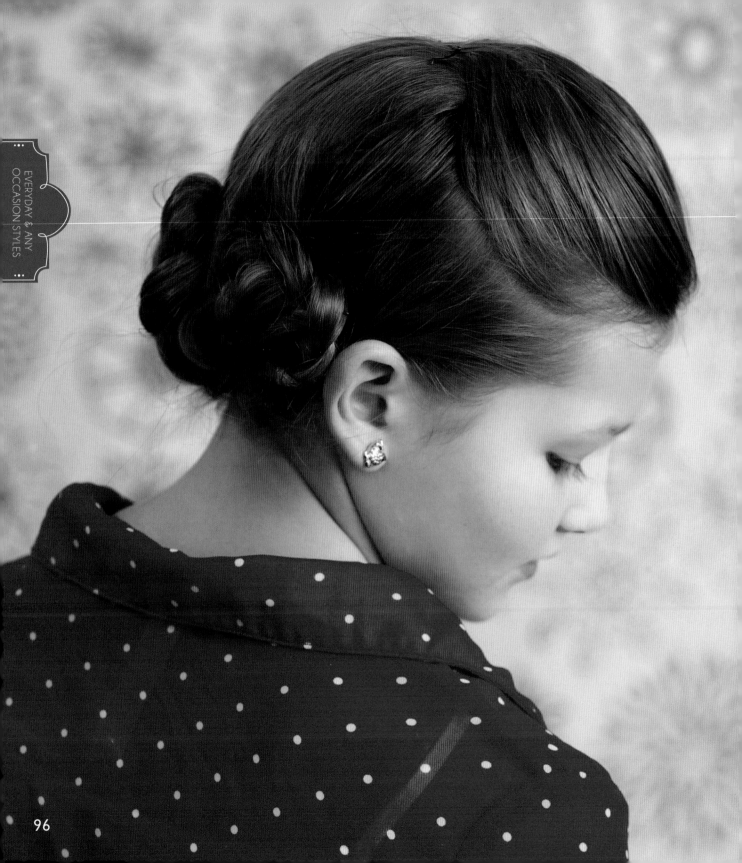

BEAUTIFUL BRAIDED BUNS

1
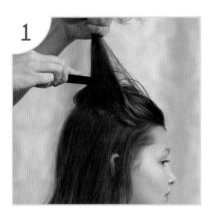

STEP 1 Slightly back comb the hair on top of the head and the crown area for added volume.

2
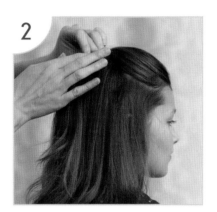

STEP 2 With this same section of hair carefully comb the top layer to make it smooth. Be careful not to comb out the teased hair underneath. Draw the hair back at each temple to make a slight bouffant or poof.

3
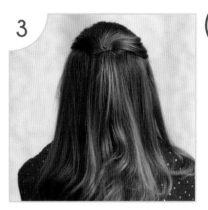

STEP 3 Secure the hair with a couple bobby pins, forming an X to make it secure.

4
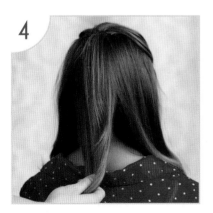

STEP 4 Divide the hair into three sections. Don't make any defined parts, just separate the sections with your hands.

5
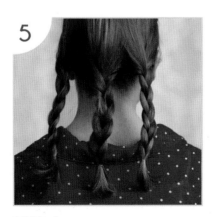

STEP 5 Starting on the right side, plait a regular 3-strand braid as shown on page 22 in each section. Secure the end of each braid with a hair elastic.

6
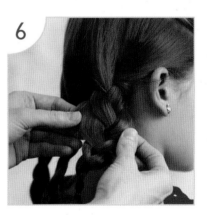

STEP 6 Pancake each braid to loosen them up a bit and make them appear wider. This is especially helpful if the hair you are working with is thin.

97

EVERYDAY & ANY
OCCASION STYLES

7

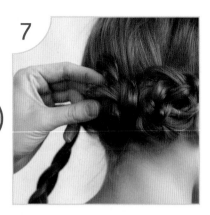

8

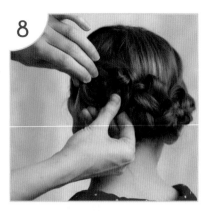

STEP 7 Starting on the right, wrap the first braid up into a bun and secure with bobby pins as needed. If the hair you are working with is shorter, don't wrap the bun too tightly or it will appear "knobby." Move to the middle braid and wrap it into a bun. Try to wrap it so it touches the edge of the braid on the right.

STEP 8 Wrap the bun on the left into a third bun and secure with bobby pins. Try to have the edge of it touch the bun in the middle to avoid a gap between them. Mist entire hairstyle with hair spray.

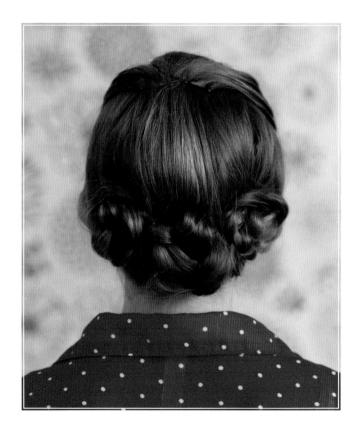

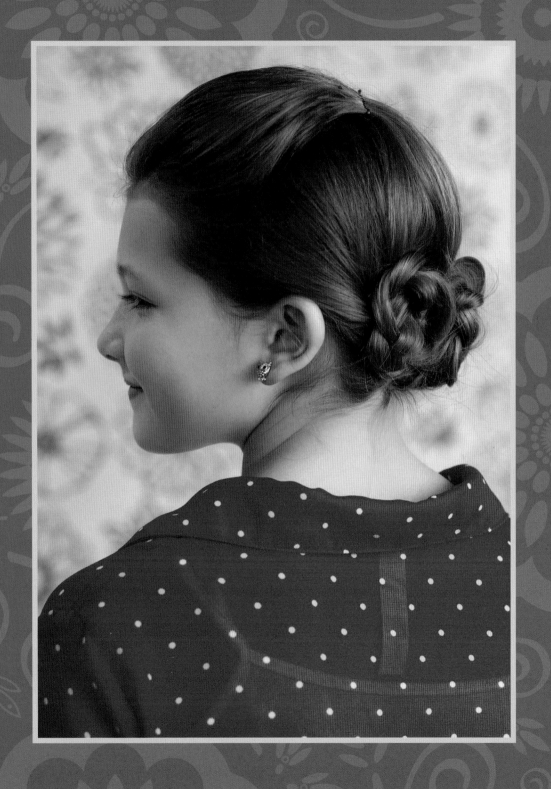

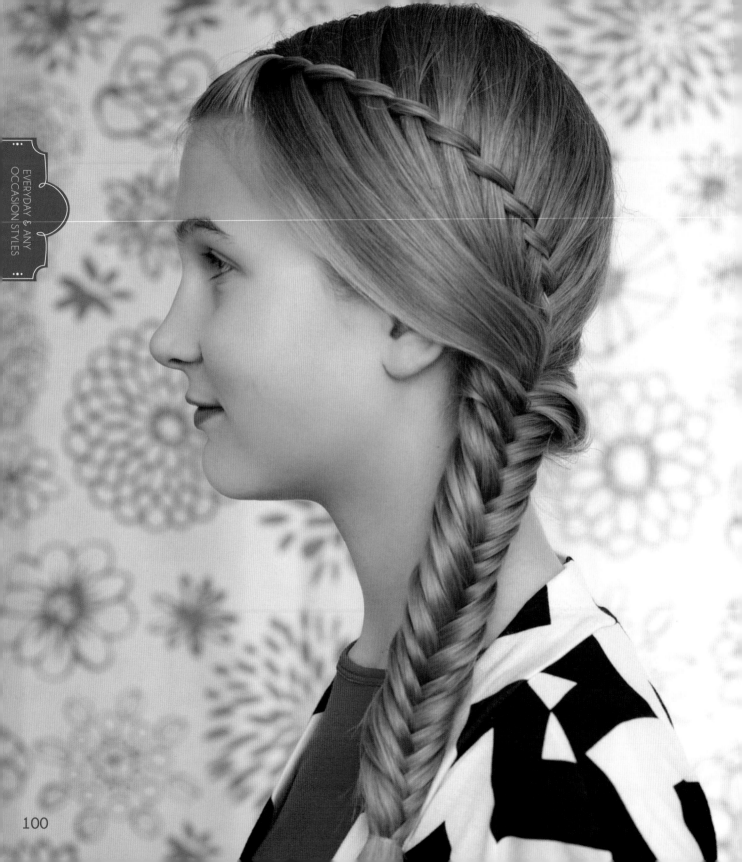

WATERFALL TWIST & FISHBONE

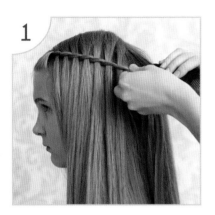

STEP 1 Make an off-center part on the right side of the head back to the crown. On the left side of the head above the left eyebrow start a waterfall twist (see page 18).

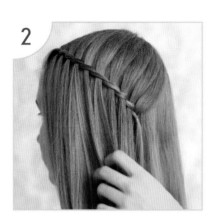

STEP 2 Add hair into the waterfall twist until you have passed the left ear and are toward the middle of the back of the head. Make sure you angle the twist so it slopes downward. Secure the twist with a clear elastic.

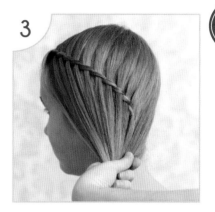

STEP 3 Gather all the hair to the left side of the head slightly over the left ear.

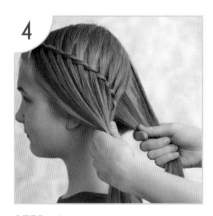

STEP 4 Divide the hair into two sections.

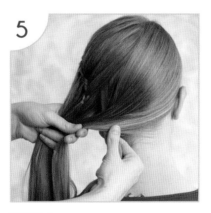

STEP 5 Proceed to make a fishbone braid as shown on page 20. Take a section of hair from the far right side of the right section of hair. Cross it over and add it to the left side.

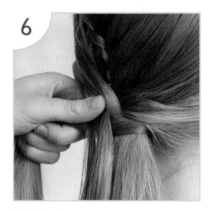

STEP 6 Repeat on the left side, taking a small section from the far left side of the left section of hair, and cross it over and add it to the right section of hair.

NOTE: Try to hold the hair tightly so the fishbone braid starts close to where the waterfall twist elastic is. If needed, slide the elastic down a bit to hide it in the start of the fishbone.

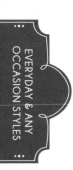

7

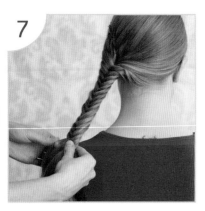

STEP 7 Continue braiding until you reach the end of the hair. Secure the fishbone braid with an elastic. Mist entire hairstyle with hair spray.

BONUS STYLES

FOR ADDITIONAL WAYS to wear this hairstyle, pull on edges of fishbone braid to pancake it and mess up the fishbone braid, or wrap the fishbone into a bun.

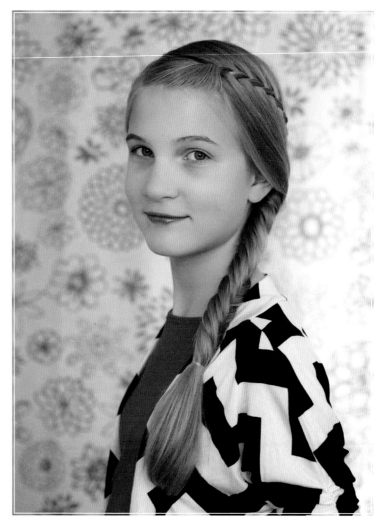

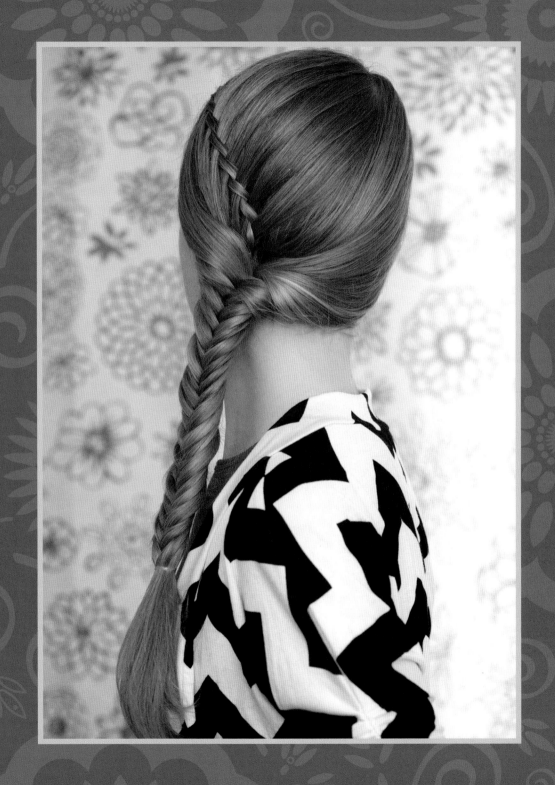

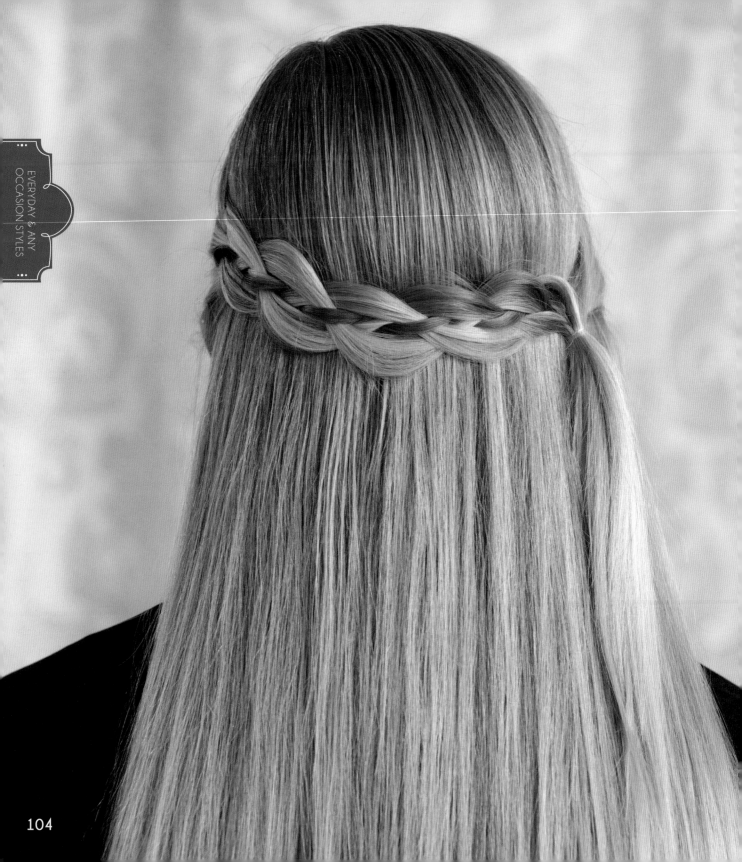

4-STRAND BRAID WRAP

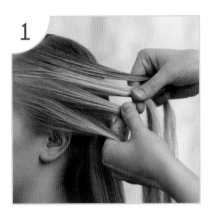

STEP 1 Part the hair on the left side back to the crown. Then part from the crown down to the left ear. Divide this section of hair into four pieces.

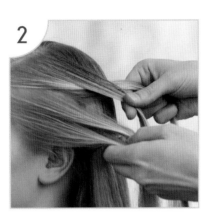

STEP 2 Begin making a 4-strand braid, as shown on page 32. Take strand 4 on the far right and cross it over strand 3.

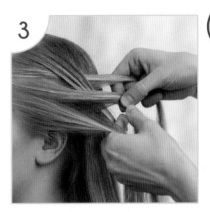

STEP 3 Pass strand 4 under strand 2.

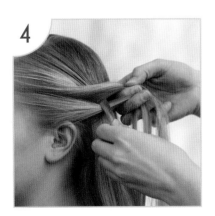

STEP 4 Then take strand 1 under what is now strand 2 (previously strand 4) and over strand 3.

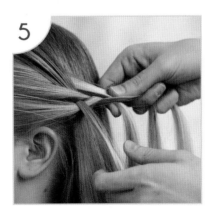

STEP 5 Continue plaiting the braid as shown on page 32.

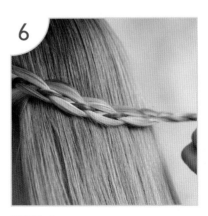

STEP 6 Make the braid long enough that it will reach around to the right side of the head.

7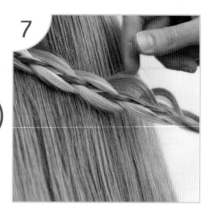

8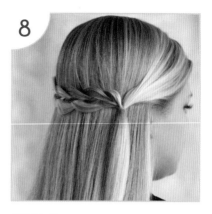

STEP 7 Starting from the bottom of the braid, gently pull on the outer edges of the braid to make it wider. Pancake as much as desired. Or, as shown on page 32, slide the strands up and back down to create a circular look around the one strand.

STEP 8 Take a section of hair on the right side near the ear and join it together with the braid. Secure with a hair elastic. You can braid this side if you desire, or just leave it straight as shown. Mist entire hairstyle with hair spray.

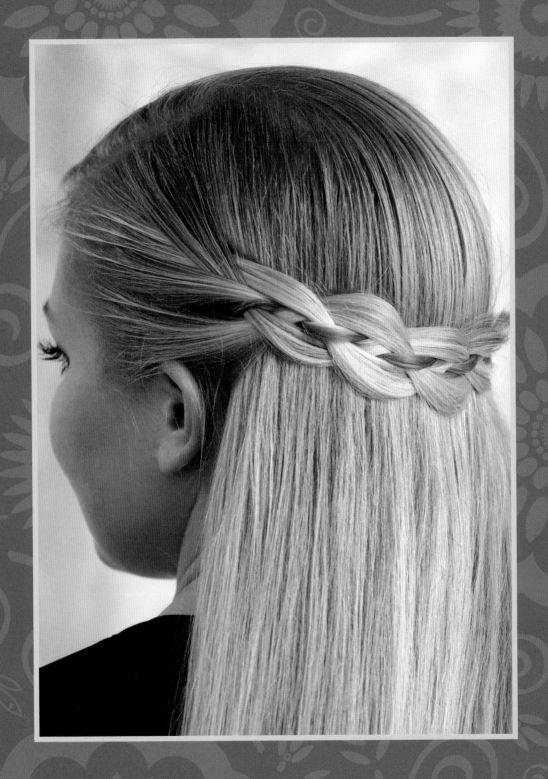

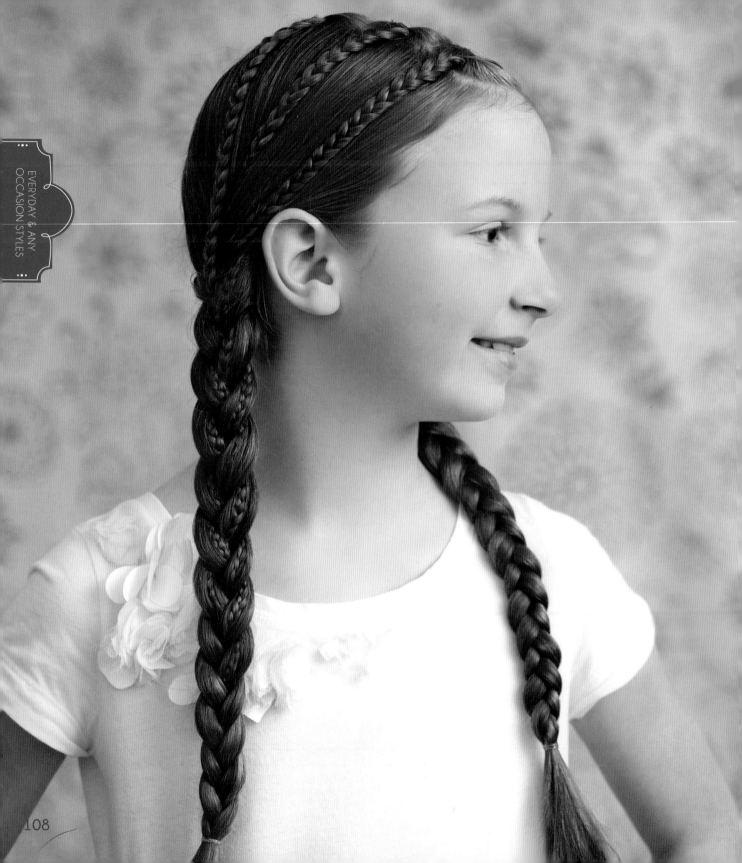

PRETTY POCAHONTAS 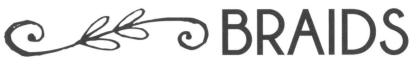 BRAIDS

At our house, we like to refer to braids on each side of the head with a part down the middle as "Pocahontas Braids." And as much as people do these, there are so many ways to make them cuter. Forget just two plain braids—add something more to make them unique.

1

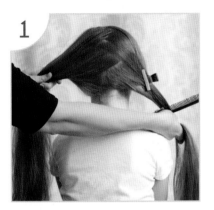

STEP 1 On the left side of the head, starting at the hairline back to the crown, make an off-center part. Then for added flair, branching off that part at the crown, make a zigzag part down the back of the head to the nape of the neck.

2

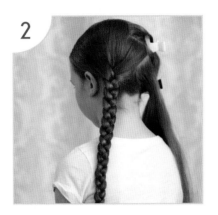

STEP 2 Gather all the hair on the left side of the head and plait a regular 3-strand braid (as shown on page 22). Braid all the way down and secure the end with a hair elastic.

3

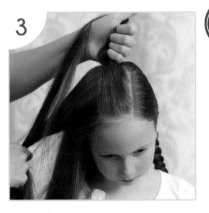

STEP 3 Make another part back to the crown that runs parallel to the off-center part. You will then have a long rectangular section of hair that is about two inches wide on the top of the head.

4

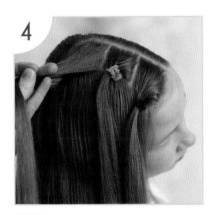

STEP 4 Divide the rectangular section into three equal sections of hair and temporarily secure them with claw clips.

5

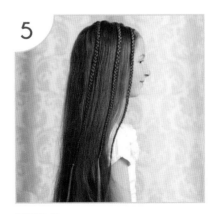

STEP 5 Plait a regular 3-strand braid in each section of hair from step 4. Secure each of them at the end with a hair elastic.

6

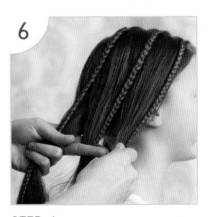

STEP 6 Gather all the straight hair on the right side and divide into 3 sections to prepare to make a 3-strand braid. Lay a micro braid on top of each section to incorporate them into this braid.

109

7

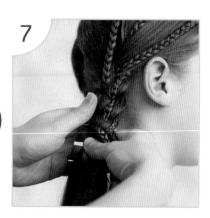

8

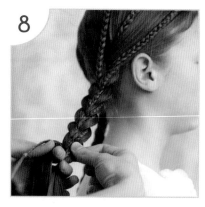

STEP 7 Begin plaiting a 3-strand braid. To get the hair to lay the best, start by crossing the right section of hair and its micro braid (the one closest to the face), over the middle section first. Then cross the left section (closest to the back of the head) over the middle.

STEP 8 Continue the normal braiding process. Be sure to keep the micro braids on top of the straight hair so they continue to show up as you braid. The micro braids may be shorter than the big braid, but just continue plaiting the braid as far down as desired. Secure the end with a hair elastic. Mist finished style with hair spray.

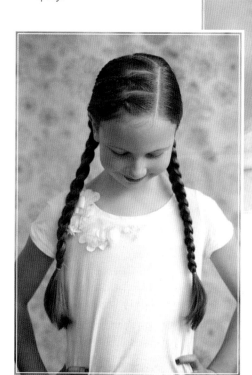

BONUS STYLES

SWITCH THE LOOK of this style up by adding rope braids in step 5, or a combo of braids and twists. You could also wind the long braids up into buns for an additional look.

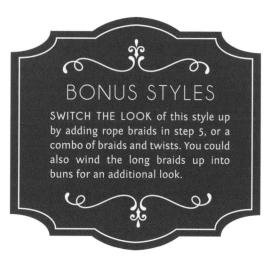

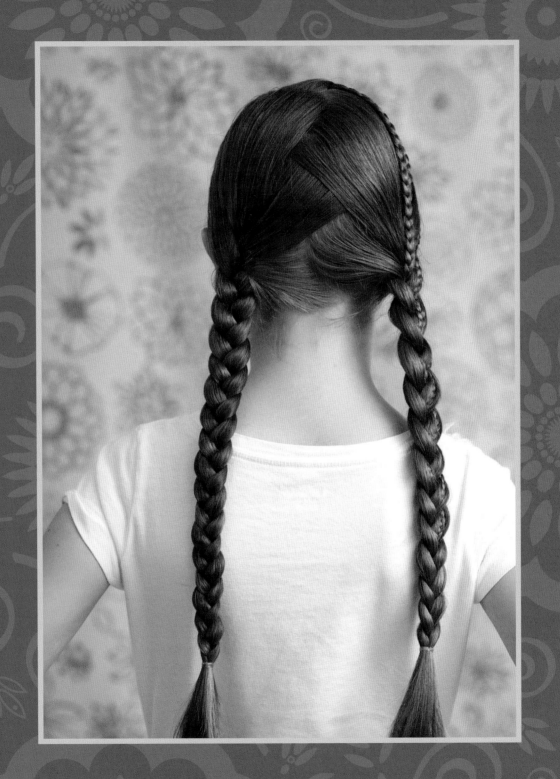

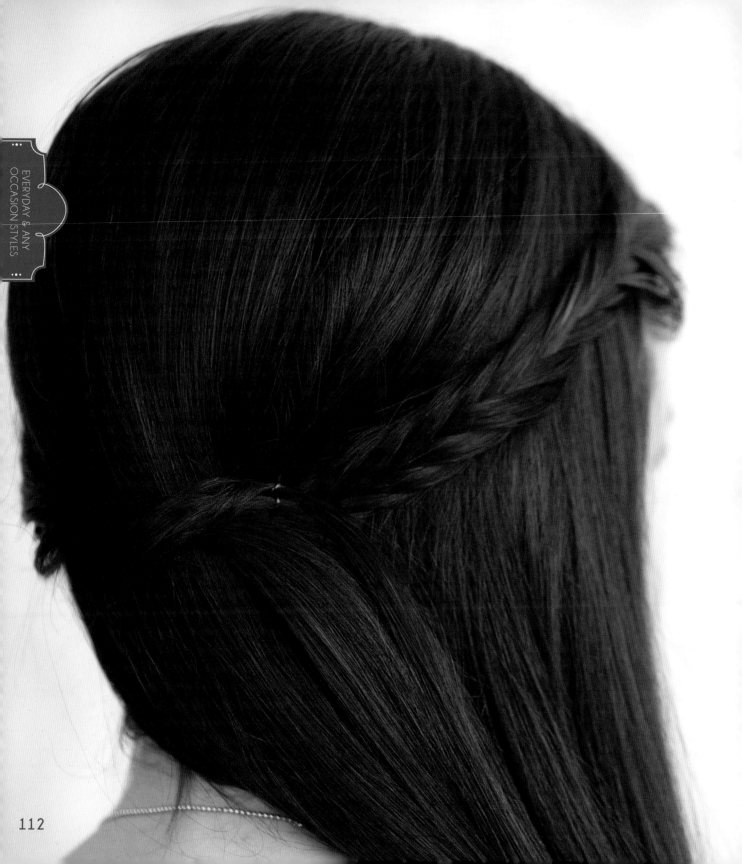

SIDESWEPT FISHBONE BRAID

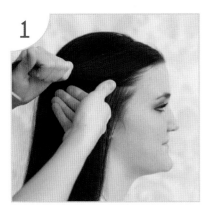

STEP 1 Make a part on the left side of the head. Section out hair from along the hairline down to the right temple.

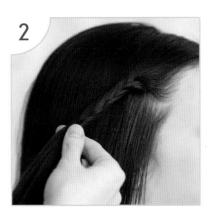

STEP 2 Divide the hair into two pieces and proceed to make a small fishbone braid as shown on page 20.

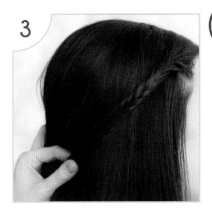

STEP 3 Continue making the fishbone braid until it can reach around the back of the head to the nape of the neck.

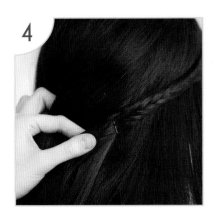

STEP 4 Secure the end of the fishbone braid into the hair with a few bobby pins.

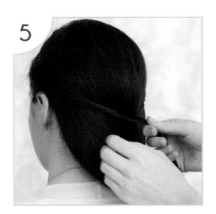

STEP 5 On the left side of the head, part out a section of hair that runs from the side part down past the left ear. Draw it backward around the back of the head and slightly twist it inward.

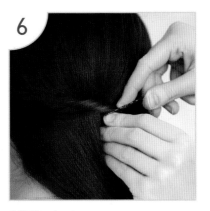

STEP 6 Anchor the twisted hair with a bobby pin just over the spot where the fishbone braid stops. Push the bobby pin in toward the left so it hides in the twist.

113

7

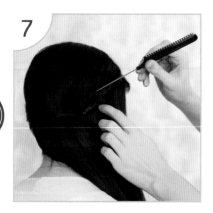

STEP 7 If desired, gently pull on the edges of the fishbone braid or use the end of a rat-tail comb to pancake it slightly. Sweep all the remaining loose hair to the side over the right shoulder. Mist entire hairstyle with hair spray.

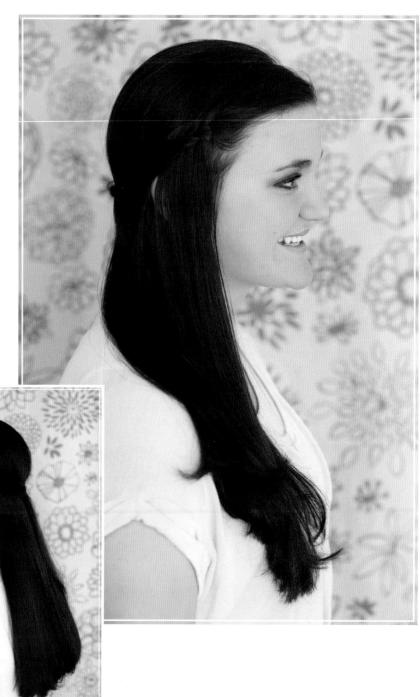

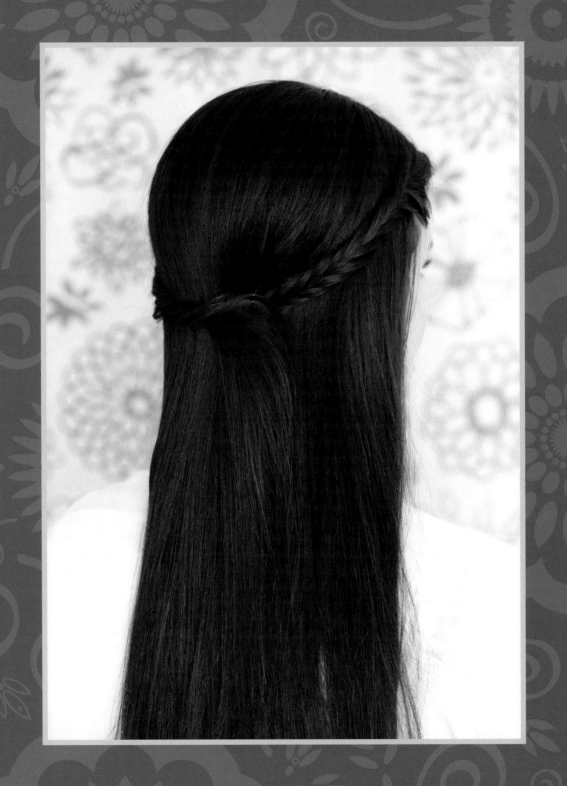

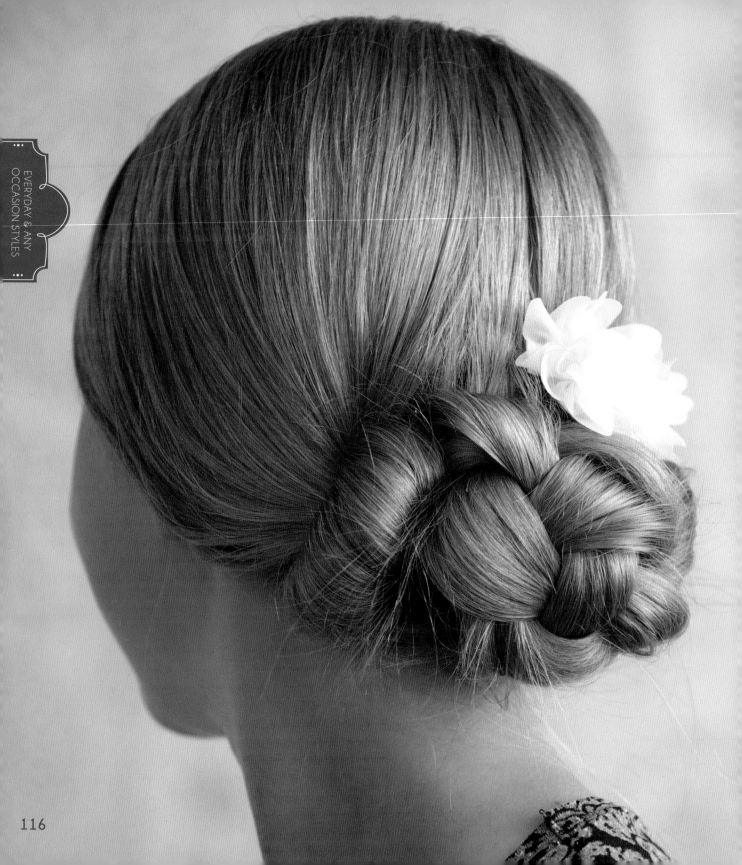

BRAIDED CHIGNON

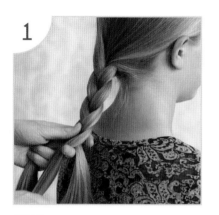

STEP 1 Divide all the hair into three even sections of hair and create a regular 3-strand braid (see page 22). Try to keep the braid fairly loose. Braid as far down as you can and secure the end with an elastic.

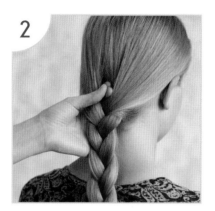

STEP 2 Above the braid take your fingers and create a hole through the hair. You can also use a Topsy Tail for this step.

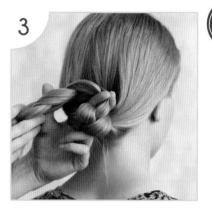

STEP 3 Draw the end of the braid up to where you have made the hole. Using your fingers, pull the braid through the hole and back down so you have flipped the braid.

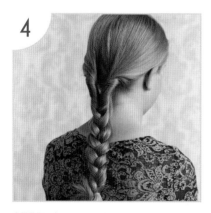

STEP 4 Repeat this one more time, flipping the braid through the hole a second time. The hair above the braid should be quite twisted and the braid will have tightened up a bit.

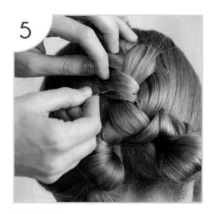

STEP 5 Flip the braid up onto the back of the head for a moment. About an inch up the braid, slide bobby pins into each side to secure the braid to the back of the head.

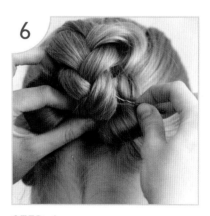

STEP 6 Draw the end of the braid back down and tuck the elastic and tail up underneath to hide it. Secure the tail and braid with bobby pins as needed.

7A

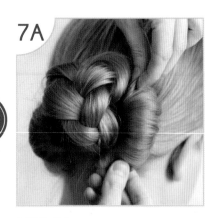

7B

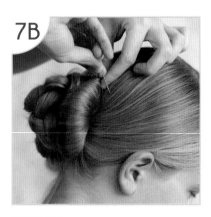

8

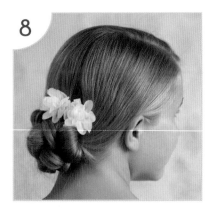

STEP 7A On both sides of the braid you will have twisted hair from flipping the ponytail in steps 3–6. Gently pull on the edges of the twisted hair so it is even with the top and bottom of the braid

STEP 7B Secure with bobby pins as needed. Do this to both sides.

STEP 8 Arrange hair until desired look is achieved. Add a flower or other accessory to dress up the style even further. Mist entire hairstyle with hair spray.

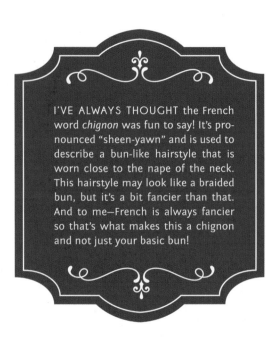

I'VE ALWAYS THOUGHT the French word *chignon* was fun to say! It's pronounced "sheen-yawn" and is used to describe a bun-like hairstyle that is worn close to the nape of the neck. This hairstyle may look like a braided bun, but it's a bit fancier than that. And to me—French is always fancier so that's what makes this a chignon and not just your basic bun!

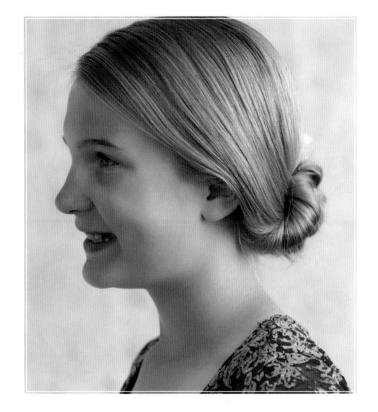

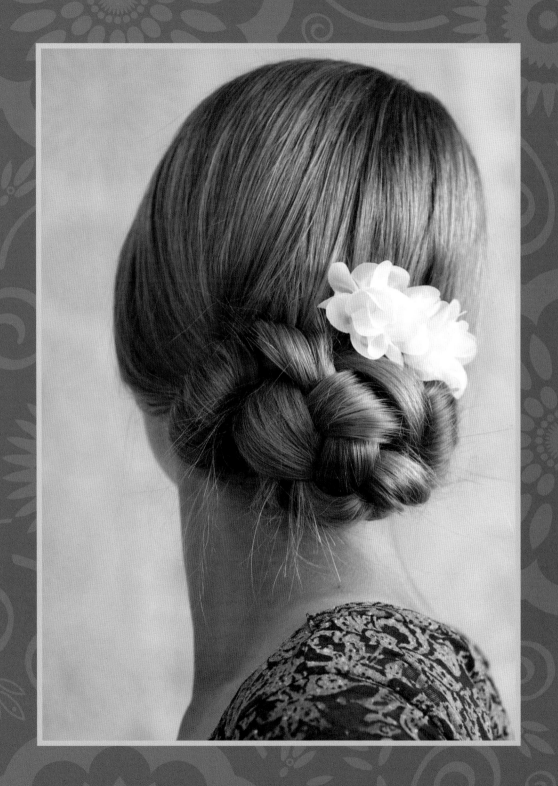

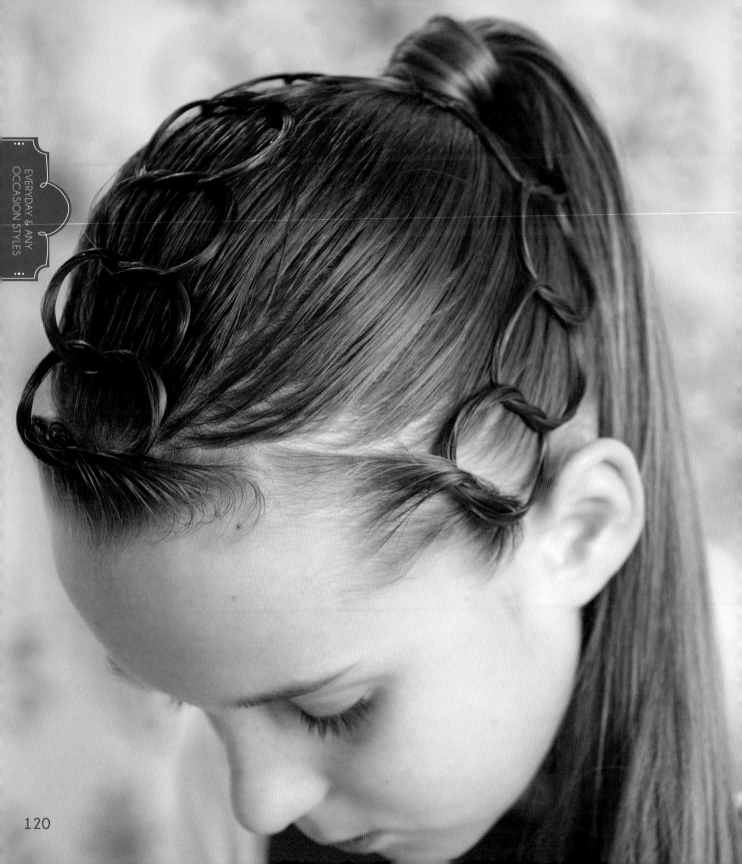

TRI-CHAIN PONYTAIL

Remember when making the chains to work with damp hair. It will create a much more defined and clean look. If you have bangs, just start the chains behind them.

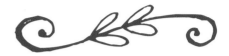

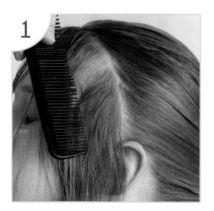

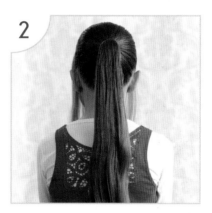

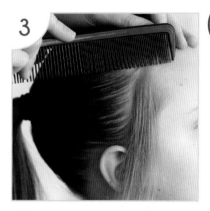

STEP 1 Make a part from the tip of the left ear over the top of the head and over to the tip of the right ear. This sections out a very small amount of hair around the whole face.

STEP 2 With all the remaining hair behind the part, gather it in the back to make a ponytail. Secure with a ponytail holder.

STEP 3 Starting on the right side of the head, in the hair around the face, make a small part that starts just above the temple.

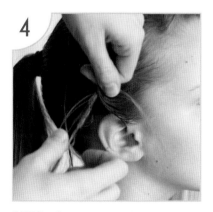

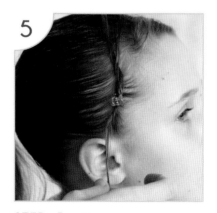

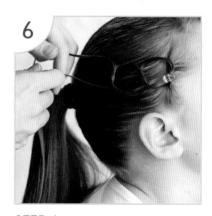

STEP 4 Mist this section of hair with water so it is rather damp. Divide the section in two pieces to begin to make a chain as shown on page 40.

STEP 5 Add a tiny claw clip to keep the start of your chain from loosening.

STEP 6 Gently take the two sections of hair and proceed to make a chain as shown on page 40. Make the circles of hair as small or big as preferred.

7

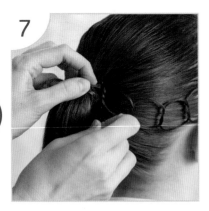

8

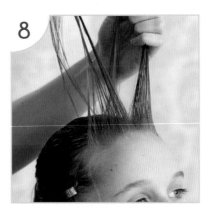

9

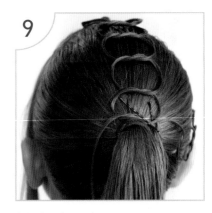

STEP 7 Make as many circles in the chain as needed until it reaches the ponytail. Temporarily slide a bobby pin over the end of the chain near the base of the ponytail to keep it from coming undone.

STEP 8 Move to the center of the head and divide out the section of hair above the forehead. Divide this section in two pieces and repeat the process to create a chain, using a small claw clip to help hold the start of the chain.

STEP 9 Once the middle chain reaches the ponytail, use another bobby pin to briefly hold it in place.

10

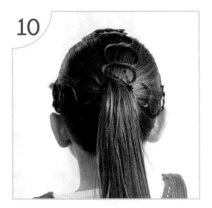

11

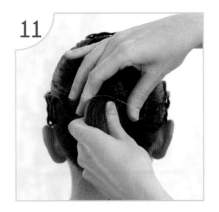

12

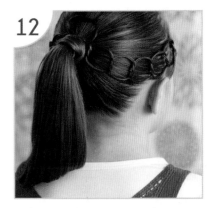

STEP 10 Repeat the process on the left side of the head with the remaining hair. Once the chain reaches the ponytail hold it in place with a bobby pin and remove the claw clips.

STEP 11 Secure all the tails from the chains to the ponytail with a clear elastic then remove the bobby pins.

STEP 12 (Optional) Wrap the base of the ponytail with hair and secure it with an elastic (see page 36). Spray entire hairstyle with hair spray.

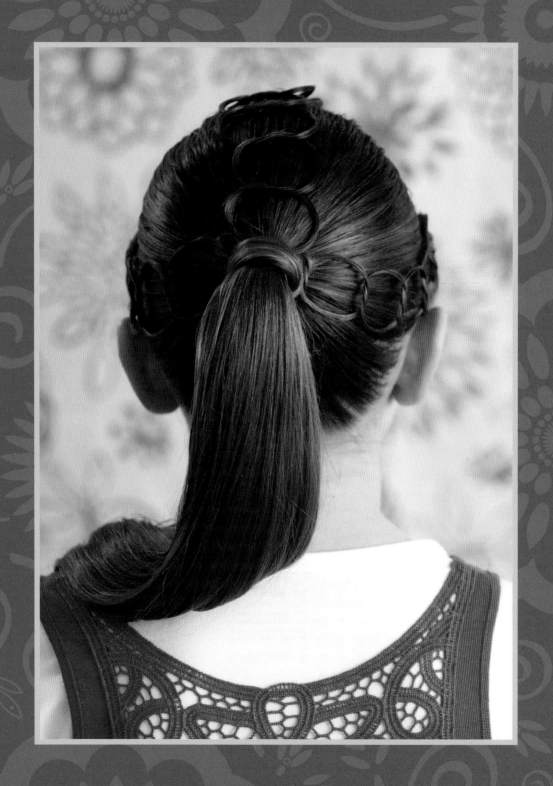

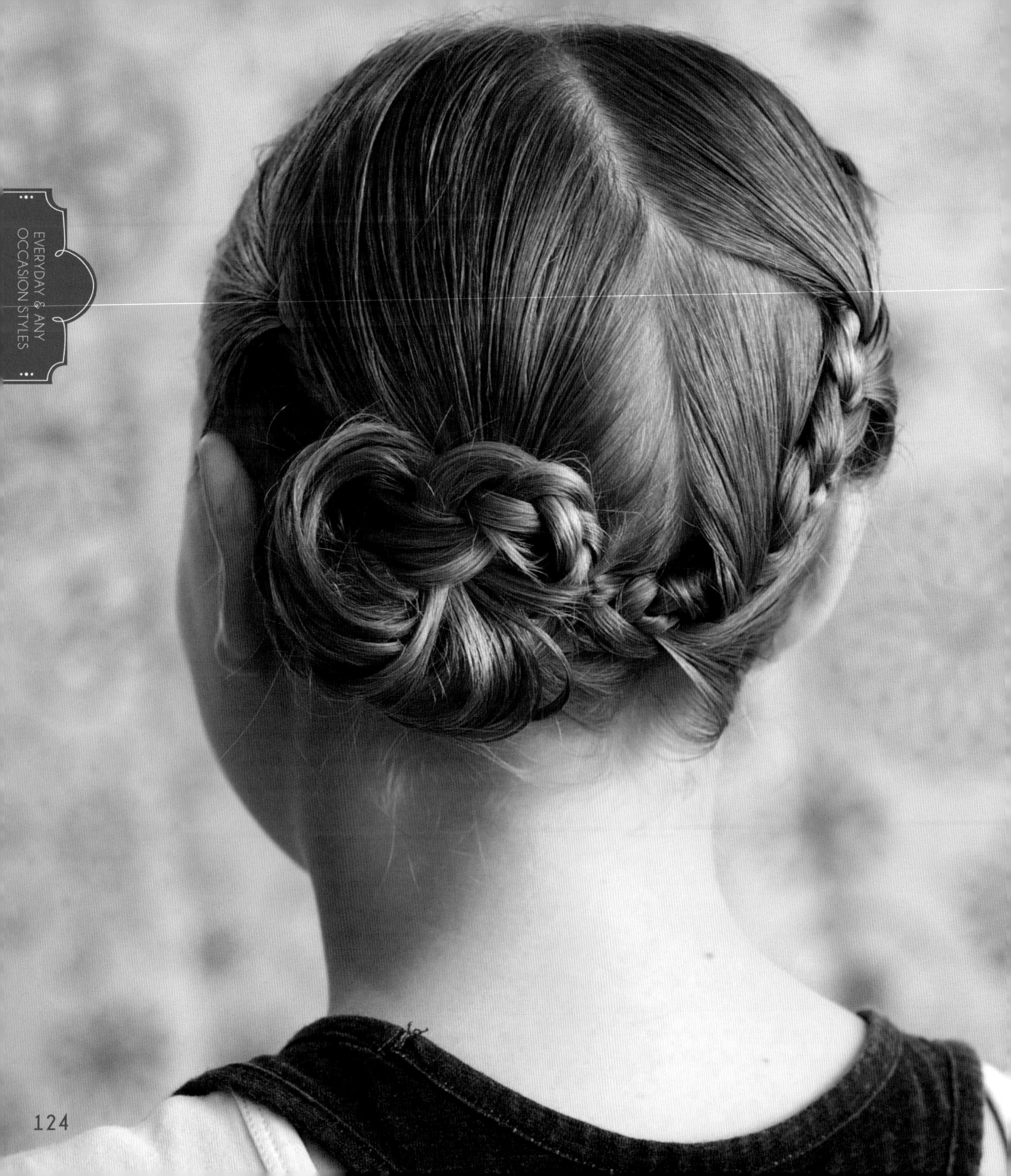

NESTED BRAIDS & BUN

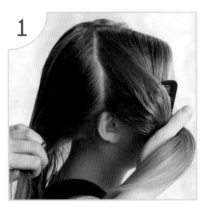

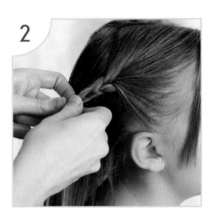

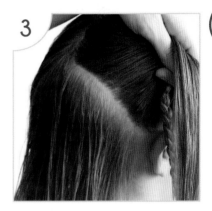

STEP 1 Make a part through the middle of the hair from the forehead to the nape of the neck. Then from the crown, make a part down to the top of the right ear.

STEP 2 Plait a regular 3-strand braid (see page 22) with this section of hair. Braid as far down as possible and secure temporarily with a small clip.

STEP 3 Part out another section of hair right behind the first one. Make the part branch off the center part and end behind the right ear.

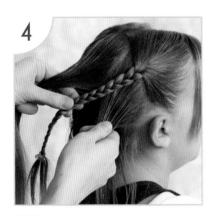

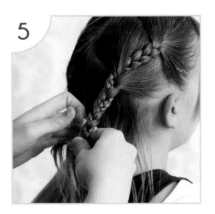

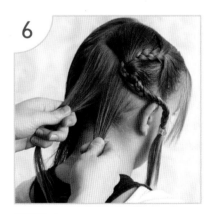

STEP 4 Divide that section of hair in half. Draw the braid from the section in front into the middle of those two pieces. Be sure to put the braid in the middle, as it will act as the middle strand for a new braid.

STEP 5 Create a new braid with this section of hair and braid as far down as possible, securing the end of with a small clip.

STEP 6 With the remaining hair on the right, repeat the same process. Divide it in half so the braid from above can be incorporated into it as the middle section.

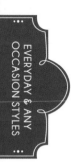

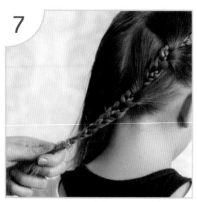

7

STEP 7 Braid all the way down and secure the end with a small clip.

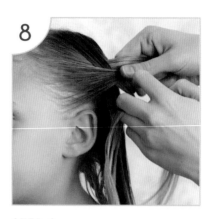

8

STEP 8 On the left side of the head, make a part from the center to the left ear. Make another 3-strand braid. Temporarily secure the end of the braid with a clip.

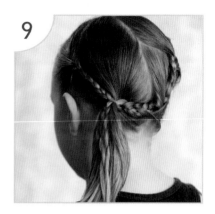

9

STEP 9 With the remaining hair on the left side of the head, comb it into a low side ponytail. Add the small braid from the left front, as well as the braid from the bottom right side. Secure all the hair with an elastic.

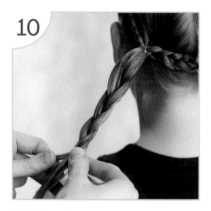

10

STEP 10 Once the ponytail has been secured remove any clips from the braids. Comb out any extra small braids that are left below the elastic. With all the hair in the ponytail, make a loose 3-strand braid and secure the end with an elastic.

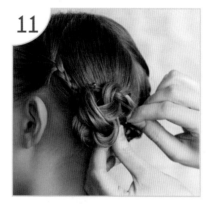

11

STEP 11 Wrap the braided ponytail in a clockwise direction to form a small bun. Secure with bobby pins as needed. Spray entire hairstyle with hair spray.

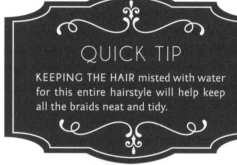

QUICK TIP

KEEPING THE HAIR misted with water for this entire hairstyle will help keep all the braids neat and tidy.

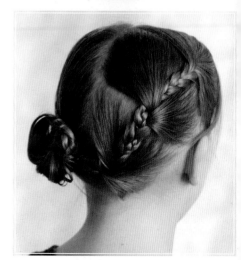

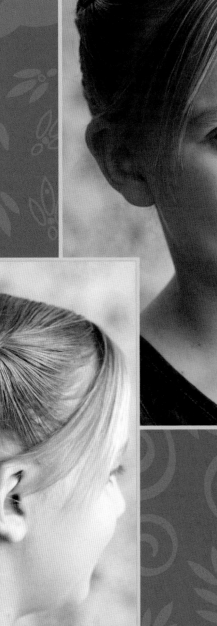

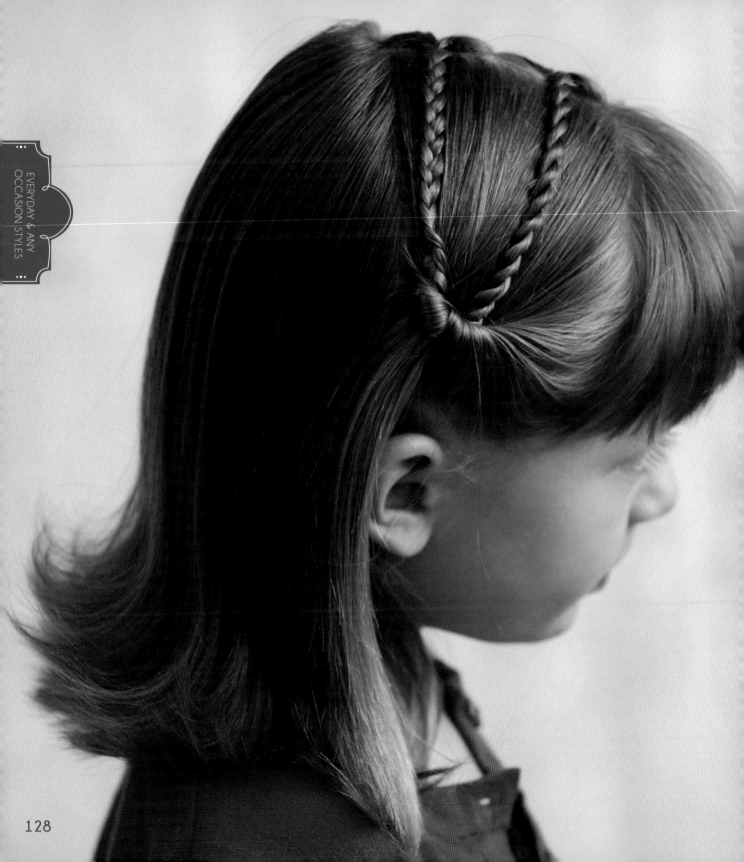

MINI BRAID & TWIST

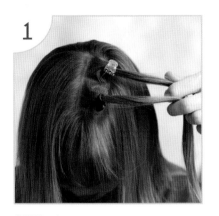

STEP 1 Create a center part that goes back to the crown. Make a second part that runs parallel to it 1 1/2-inches to the left. You will have parted out a rectangular section of hair. Divide that in half to make two small square sections.

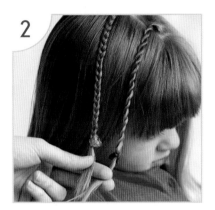

STEP 2 With the front square section make a rope braid (see page 16) and with the back square make a 3-strand braid (see page 22). Temporarily secure both of them with a small claw clip.

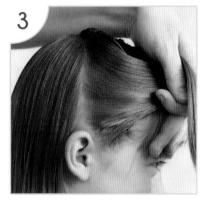

STEP 3 Flip the twist and braid out of the way to the left side of the head for the moment. Make a part from the crown down to the right ear.

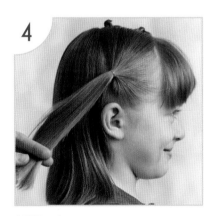

STEP 4 With that section of hair make a small ponytail slightly above the right ear. Secure it with a hair elastic.

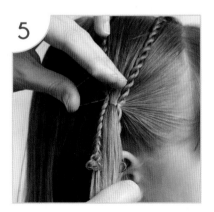

STEP 5 Bring the twist and braid back over the head and with another elastic, secure them to the ponytail you created in Step 4. Remove the small claw clips.

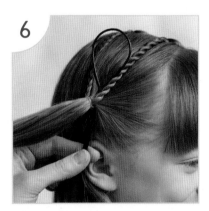

STEP 6 If needed, loosen the ponytail slightly. Place the pointed end of a Topsy Tail in between the twist and braid and behind the elastic. Push the pointed end through the hair so it sits below the ponytail.

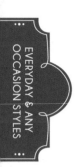

EVERYDAY & ANY OCCASION STYLES

7

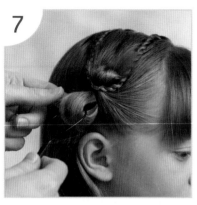

8

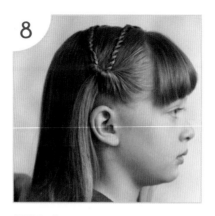

STEP 7 As shown on page 34, place the ponytail through the looped end of the Topsy Tail and flip the ponytail.

STEP 8 Comb through the flipped ponytail to smooth out the hair, and if desired, curl the ends of all the hair in back. Mist entire hairstyle with hair spray.

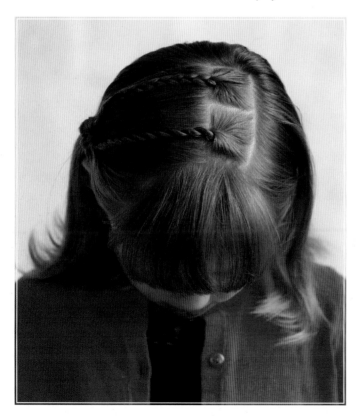

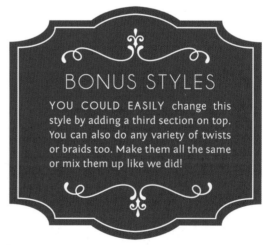

BONUS STYLES

YOU COULD EASILY change this style by adding a third section on top. You can also do any variety of twists or braids too. Make them all the same or mix them up like we did!

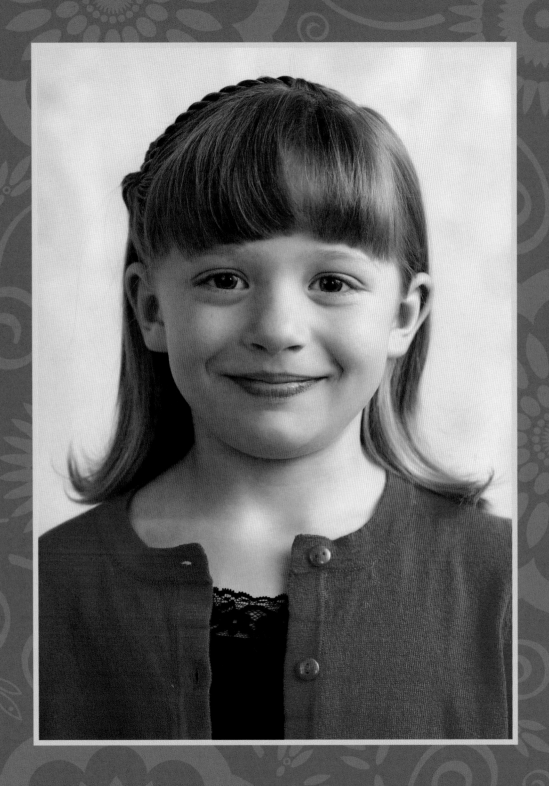

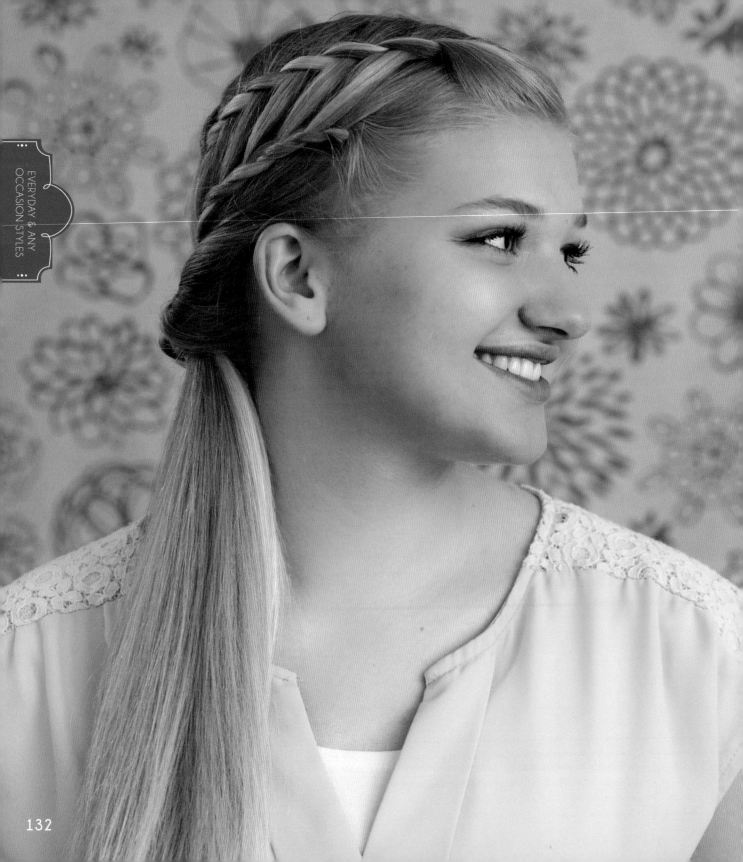

LADDER BRAID FLIPPED PONYTAIL

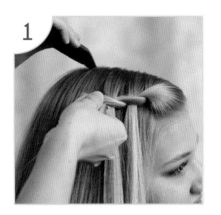

STEP 1 Make a part on the left side of the head back to the crown. On the right side of the part, create a waterfall twist, as shown on page 18.

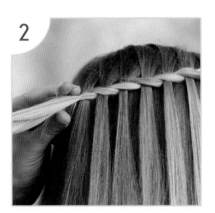

STEP 2 Once the waterfall twist reaches the middle of the back of the head, stop adding hair to the twist and secure it with an elastic.

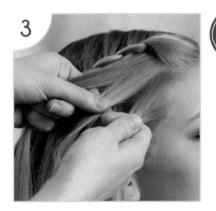

STEP 3 Right below the twist, grab the remaining hair near the face and divide it into three sections. Make one complete rotation of a braid. (Right over middle piece, left over middle piece.)

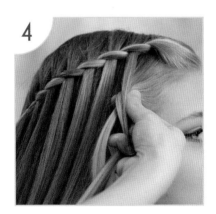

STEP 4 After you have crossed the left (top) section over the middle section of the braid, grab the first piece of hair hanging down from the twist above and add it into the braid. Remember a lace braid adds hair to just one side.

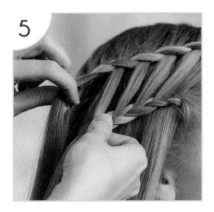

STEP 5 Continue braiding, only adding hair from the twist into the braid so it creates a ladder between the braid and twist.

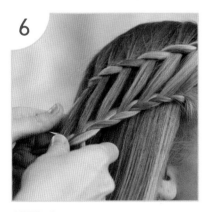

STEP 6 Stop braiding once you have no more hair from the twist to add. Secure the braid with an elastic.

133

EVERYDAY & ANY OCCASION STYLES

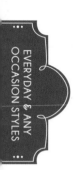

7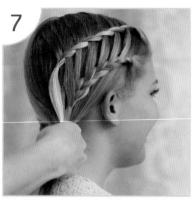

8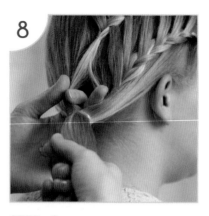

9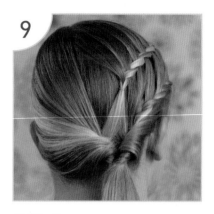

STEP 7 Gather all the hair to the right side of the neck to make a loose ponytail. Secure with an elastic.

STEP 8 Above the elastic, bring your fingers through the hair, making a hole.

STEP 9 Flip the ponytail through the hole and pull it out the bottom. This can also be done using a Topsy Tail, as shown on page 34. Mist entire hairstyle with hair spray.

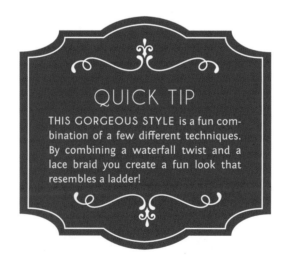

QUICK TIP

THIS GORGEOUS STYLE is a fun combination of a few different techniques. By combining a waterfall twist and a lace braid you create a fun look that resembles a ladder!

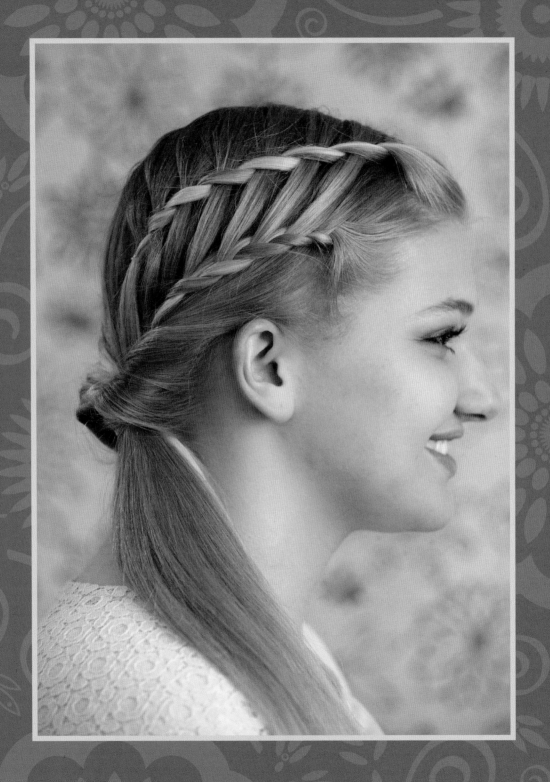

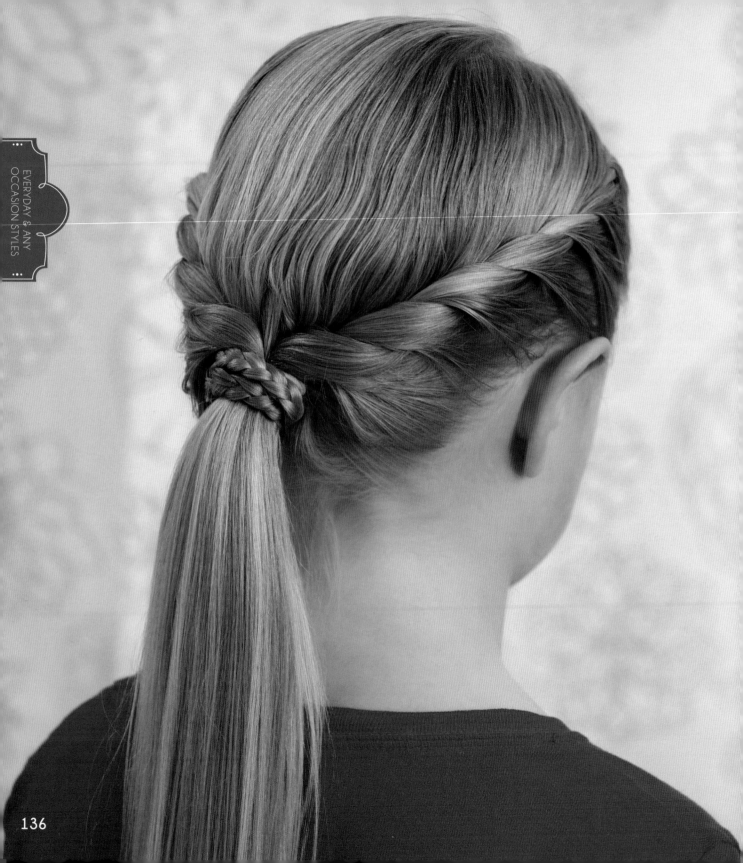

136

FRENCH ROPE TWISTS

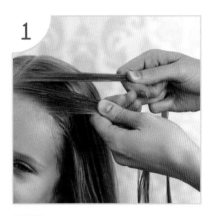

STEP 1 Make a part on the right side of the head back to the crown. Section off a small triangular section of hair along the hairline on the left side of the head. Divide that section of hair into two.

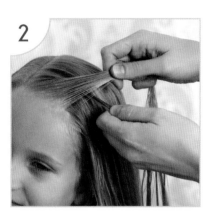

STEP 2 Cross the bottom section of hair over the top section so they change places and make an X.

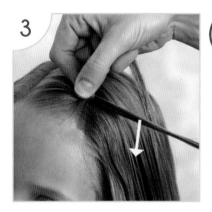

STEP 3 Drop the bottom section of hair so it lays on the rest of the hair hanging down below.

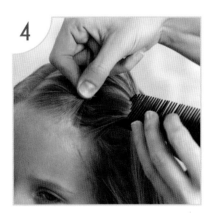

STEP 4 With a comb or your fingers, grab some hair from below and draw it upwards. Be sure to include the hair you dropped in Step 3. You may need to use your comb or fingers to smooth this section of hair.

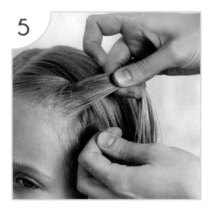

STEP 5 Pass this new thicker section of hair that was on the bottom over the thinner top section of hair so they trade places.

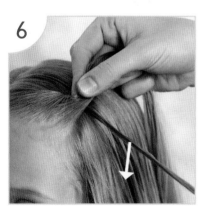

STEP 6 Now the thinner top section is on the bottom. As you did in step 3, drop the bottom section of hair so it lays on the hair below.

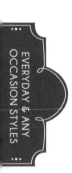

7

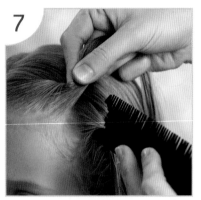

STEP 7 Once again, with a comb or your fingers, grab hair from below, and be sure to include the piece you dropped.

8

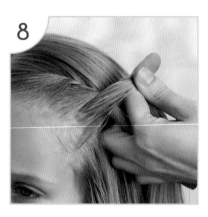

STEP 8 Cross the bottom section over the top section so they trade places.

9

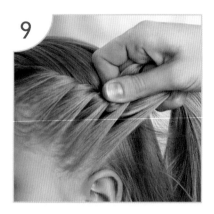

STEP 9 Continue the process of dropping and adding hair to the bottom section and crossing the bottom section over the top section so they trade places. Continue working your way along the hairline past the left ear.

10

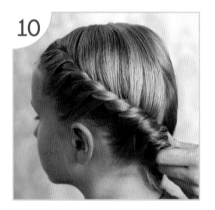

STEP 10 Once you reach the nape of the neck, stop twisting and temporarily secure the twist with a clip so it doesn't unwind.

11

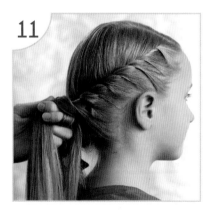

STEP 11 Repeat on the right side of the head until you run out of hair to add, and meet in the middle with the other twist.

12

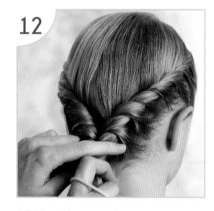

STEP 12 Combine the two twists at the middle of the neck and secure with a ponytail holder or an elastic. With a comb, smooth the hair down on the back of the head as needed.

BONUS STYLE

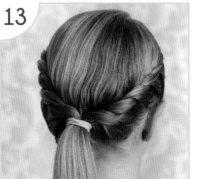

STEP 13 You can be done with this pretty style at this point and add an accessory to cover your elastic or you can finish it off with these optional steps.

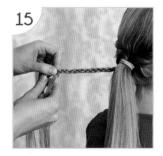

STEP 14 Take a small section of hair from underneath the ponytail and mist it with water or hair spray.

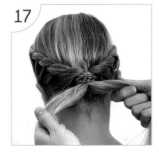

STEP 15 With this small section of hair, make a micro braid. Braid most of the way down and temporarily secure the end with a small claw clip.

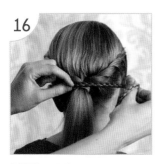

STEP 16 Wrap the micro braid around the base of the ponytail a few times, covering up the elastic at the nape of the neck. Secure the braid to the base of the ponytail with an elastic as is done in a Hair-Wrapped Ponytail (see page 36).

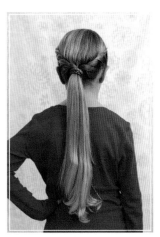

STEP 17 Cinch the ponytail if needed to hide the elastic and push the braid closer to the base of the ponytail. Add a few curls to the ends of the ponytail if desired. Mist entire hairstyle with hair spray.

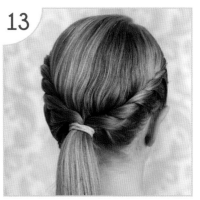

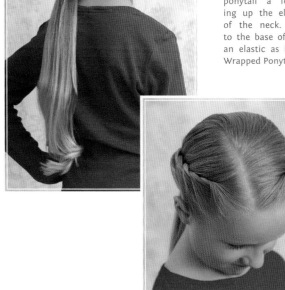

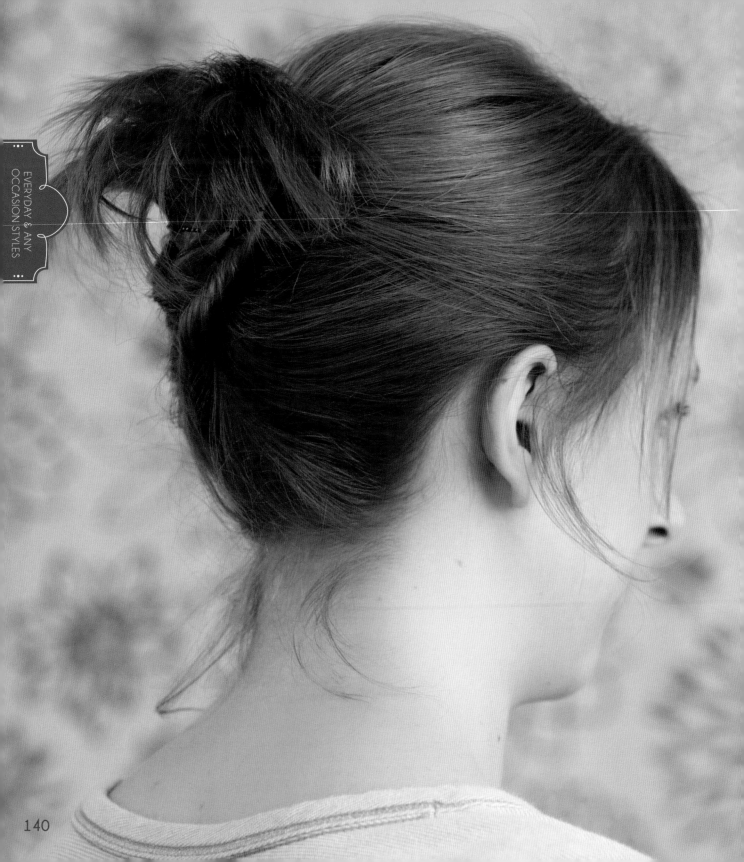

THE PEACOCK TWIST

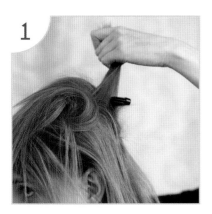

STEP 1 At the crown, back comb several sections of hair at the roots to add volume.

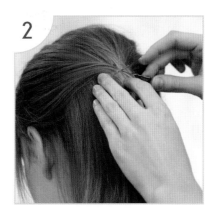

STEP 2 Flip the hair back over and smooth the top layer with a comb. Section out hair from ear to ear and make a half pony. Secure it with a few bobby pins forming an X in the middle of the back of the head.

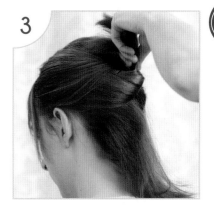

STEP 3 Section out half of the hair remaining down in back and twist it in an upward direction like you are making a French twist. Bring the twist up high enough that it covers the X of bobby pins from step 2.

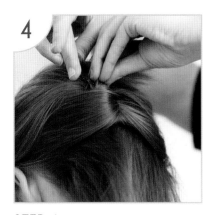

STEP 4 Hold the hair with one hand so it remains twisted and secure it with a few bobby pins with the other hand.

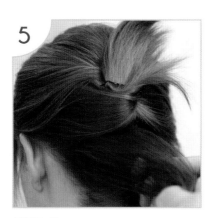

STEP 5 Allow the ends of the twist to spray upward above the bobby pins.

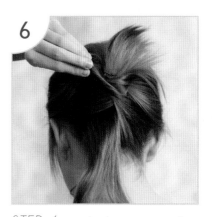

STEP 6 Divide the remaining hair in back into a left and right section. Take the right section and twist it in toward the head. Draw it upward and to the left side of the twist from step 3.

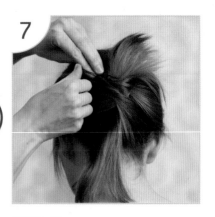

STEP 7 Secure the twist with a bobby pin on the left side of the twist made in step 3. Open the bobby pin up so it straddles the twist. Insert the bobby pin aiming the open ends downward for a better grip.

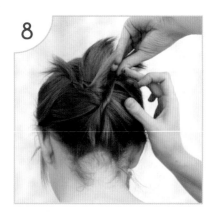

STEP 8 Take the remaining hair on the left side, twist it and draw it upward toward the right side of the head. Secure with a bobby pin.

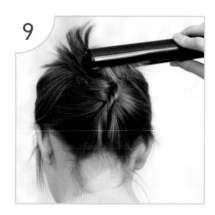

STEP 9 With a flat iron or curling iron, slightly turn under the ends of the hair spraying up.

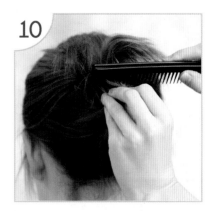

STEP 10 If needed, back comb the ends as well to give it a messier appearance. Spray the ends and entire style with finishing spray to hold this fun and funky look.

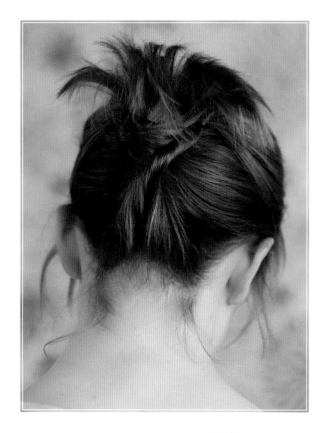

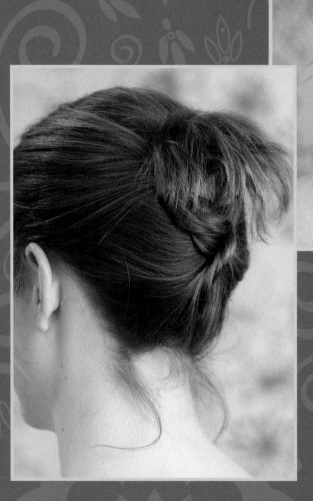

QUICK TIP

THIS STYLE CAN be done whether you have bangs or not. It's also a great style if you are growing bangs as it helps keep the hair out of the eyes during those awkward lengths.

SIDE PONY & FRENCH BRAID

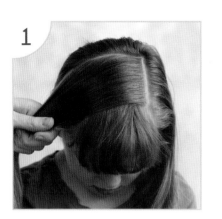

STEP 1 Make an off-center part on the left of the head back to the crown. From the crown, part down to the right ear. With all the rest of the hair in back, temporarily hold it out of the way with a clip.

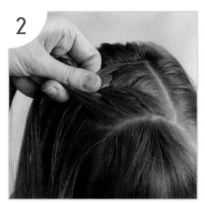

STEP 2 Starting on top of the head, begin creating a French Braid (see page 28). Add hair from both sides of the braid.

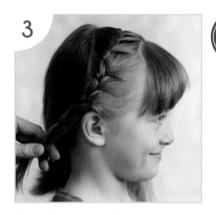

STEP 3 Add hair to the French braid until you reach the ear and then stop adding hair to the braid. Continue braiding a regular 3-strand braid until you reach the end of the hair. Use a small clip to temporarily secure the end of the braid.

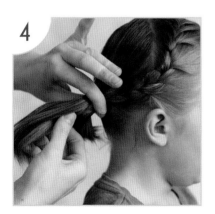

STEP 4 Draw all the remaining hair in back to the right side of the head to create a ponytail. Add the end of the braid into the ponytail and secure it all together with an elastic.

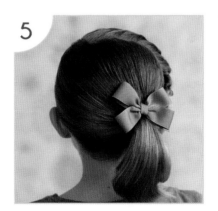

STEP 5 Smooth out any bumps in the hair and spray with finishing spray. Curl the ponytail if desired and add a cute accessory to cover the elastic.

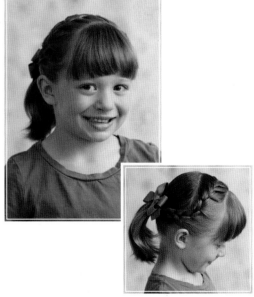

145

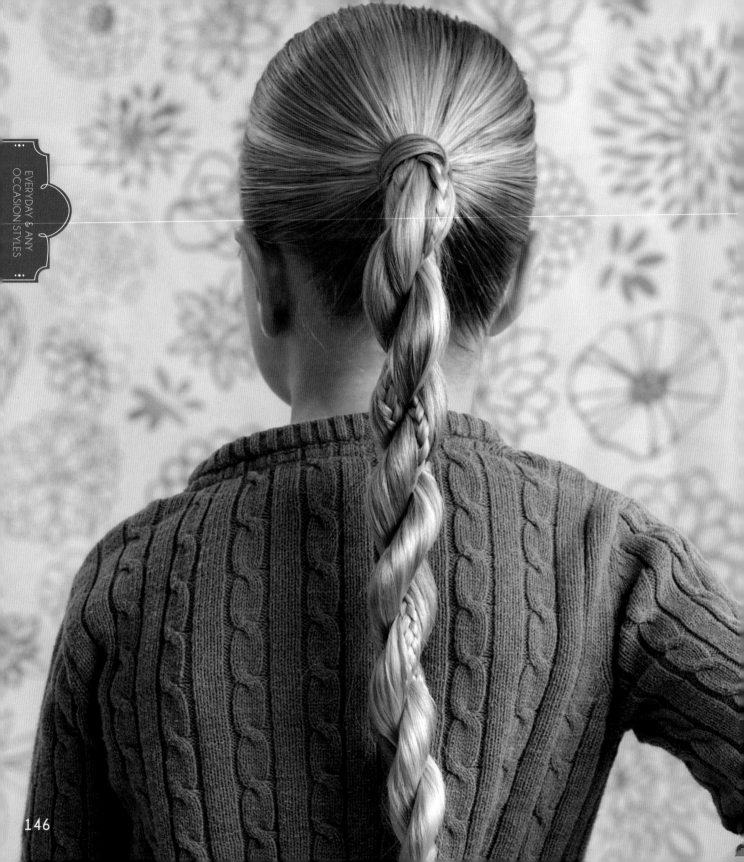

MICRO BRAIDS WITH
❦ A TWIST

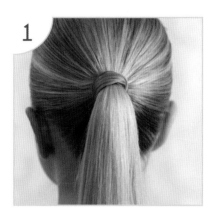

1

STEP 1 Gather all the hair into a ponytail and secure with an elastic. If you wish, cover the elastic by wrapping it with a small section of hair (as shown on page 36).

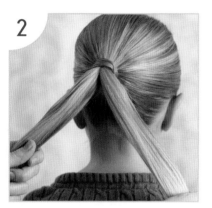

2

STEP 2 Divide the ponytail in two even sections.

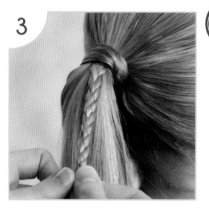

3

STEP 3 From the section of hair on the right, take a small amount of hair from the top and make a regular 3-strand braid (as shown on page 22), creating a "micro braid."

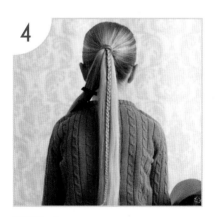

4

STEP 4 Braid all the way to the end of the hair and secure the end with an elastic.

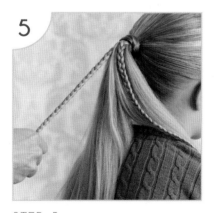

5

STEP 5 Move the micro braid and right half of the ponytail out of the way, and take a small section of hair from the top of the left side of the ponytail. Create another micro braid and secure the end with an elastic.

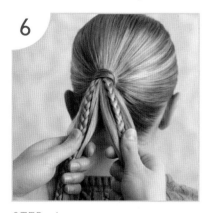

6

STEP 6 Keep the ponytail divided in half and the micro braids lying smoothly on top of the straight hair.

147

7

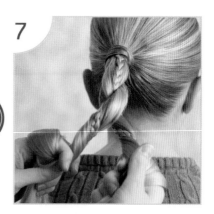

STEP 7 Make a rope braid (see page 16) twisting both sections of hair clockwise and then passing the right strand back over counterclockwise. You may need to do this slowly to ensure the micro braids stay visible and don't get buried in the straight hair. Continue twisting until you reach the bottom of the hair. Secure the end with an elastic.

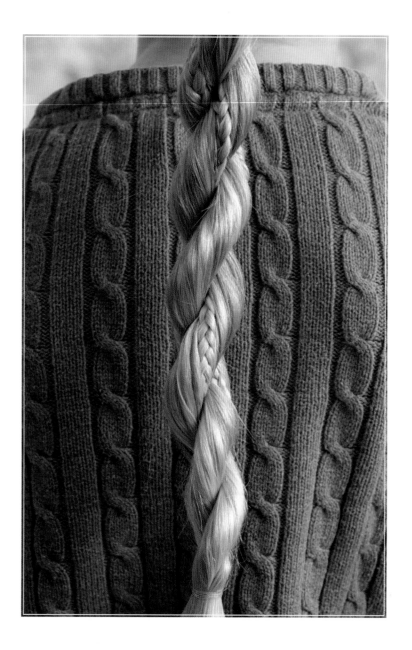

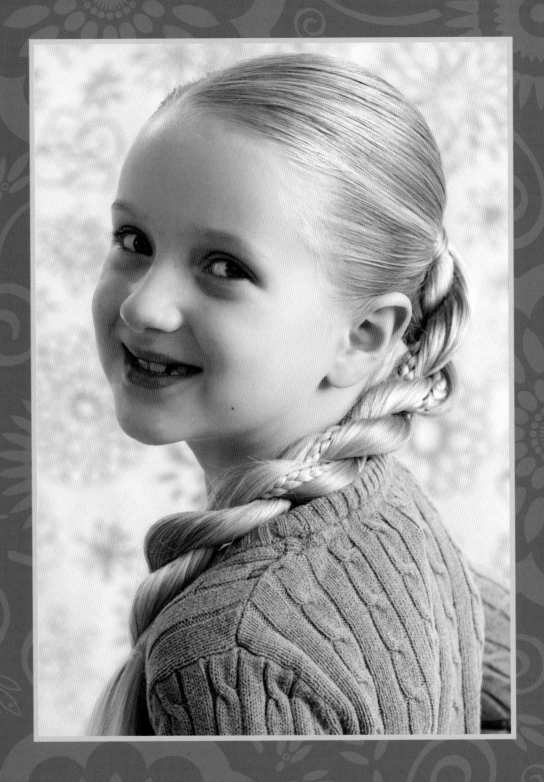

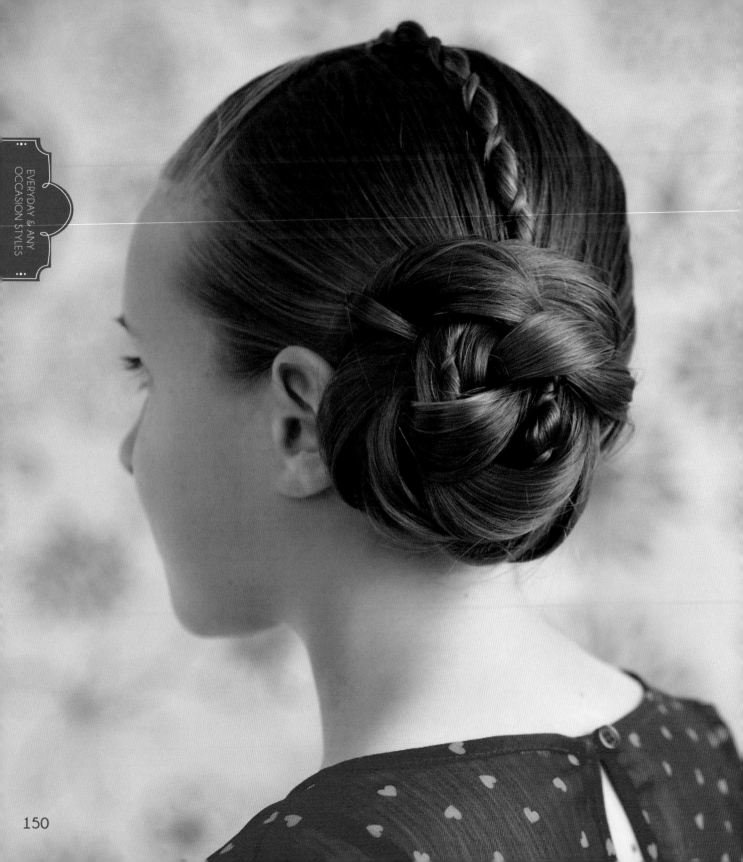

UNEVEN ROPE TWIST & BUN

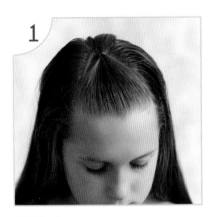

STEP 1 Make a triangular part at the front of the head and gather that hair into a small ponytail. Secure the ponytail with a clear elastic.

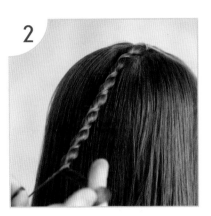

STEP 2 Divide the hair from that small ponytail into a thick and a thin section. Begin twisting to create an uneven rope twist (see page 17).

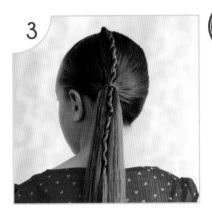

STEP 3 Twist as far down as you can and secure the end with a clear elastic. Gather all the hair, including the uneven rope twist into a ponytail behind the left ear. Secure that ponytail with an elastic.

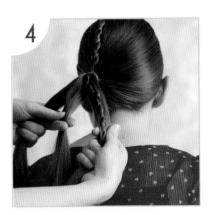

STEP 4 Divide the ponytail into three even sections. Lay the twist from above on top of the right section of hair.

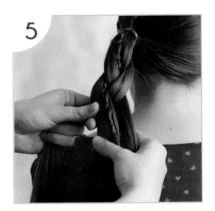

STEP 5 Loosely make a regular 3-strand braid in the ponytail. Try to keep the uneven twist on top of the hair so it shows through the braid.

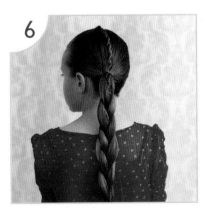

STEP 6 Continue braiding even if the twist doesn't run the entire length of the braid. Secure the end of the braid with an elastic.

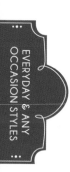

7

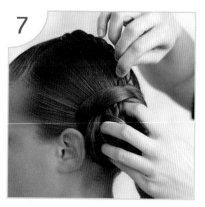

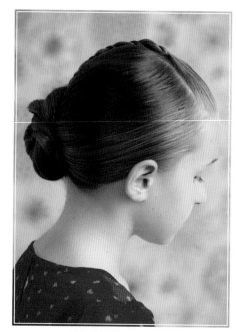

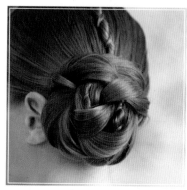

STEP 7 Draw the braid up and wrap in a clockwise direction to create a bun near the left ear. Don't wrap it too tightly so the uneven twist can be seen peeking through. Secure the bun with bobby pins as needed. Mist with holding spray.

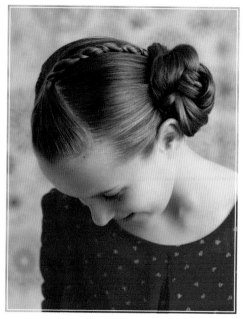

BONUS STYLES

THIS PRETTY STYLE can actually be worn three different ways. You can create the twist & join it to a pony and be finished after Step 3 creating a more casual style. You can also be done after Step 6 once you have braided the ponytail. Or of course, you can complete all 7 steps for the finished look with the hair wrapped up into a bun for a more elegant look.

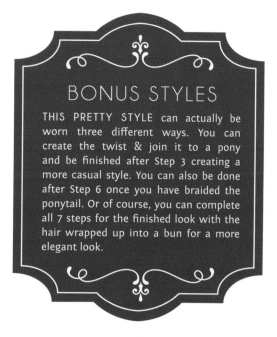

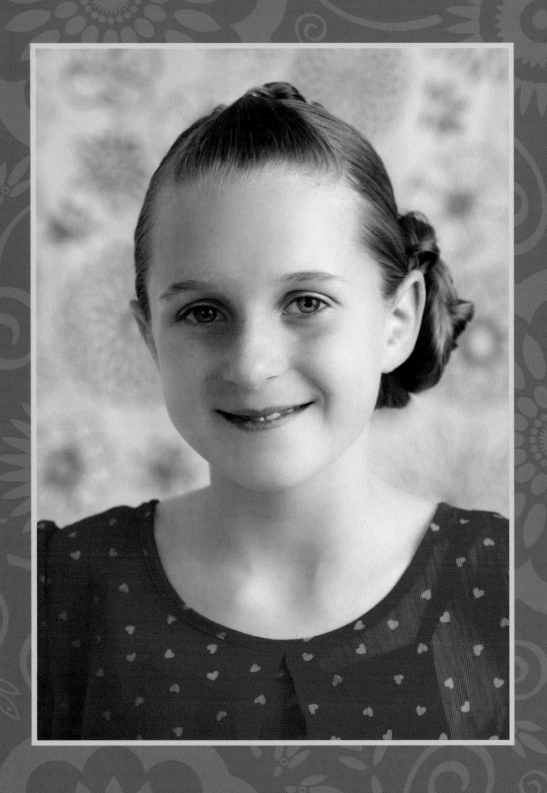

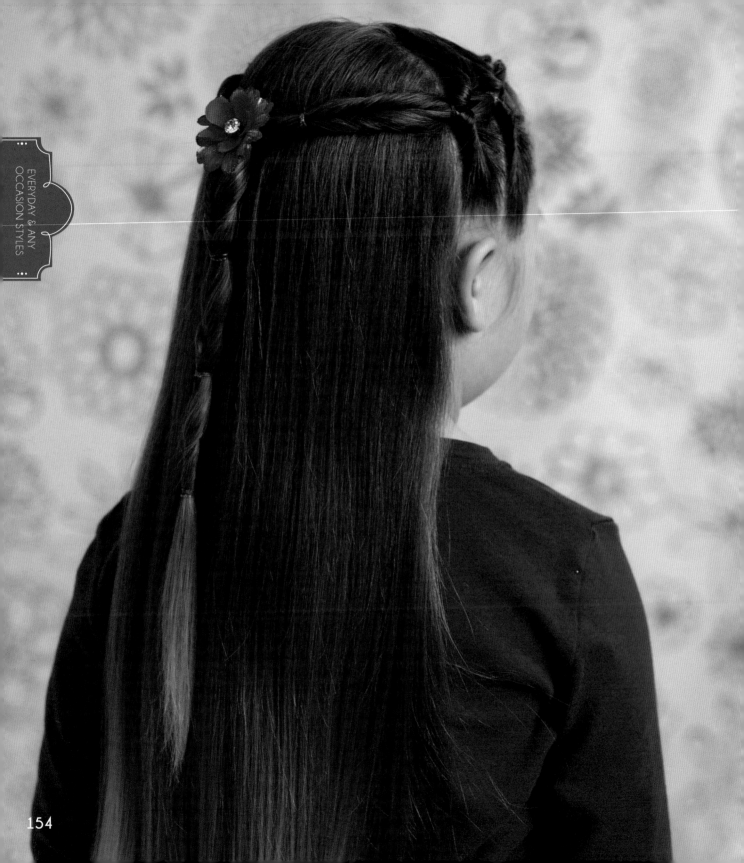

FAUX FISHBONES

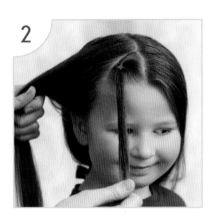

STEP 1 Part the hair right down the middle back to the crown. Then part the hair from ear to ear. Secure the hair behind the ears with a clip temporarily.

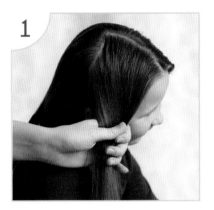

STEP 2 On the right side of the head, part out a small triangular section of hair. Make a loose ponytail with this section and secure with an elastic.

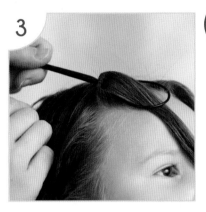

STEP 3 As shown on page 34, flip the ponytail under. Once the ponytail is flipped, if needed, cinch the flipped ponytail so it is not as loose.

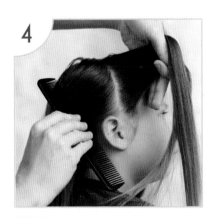

STEP 4 Branching off the center part, make another part down to the front of the right ear.

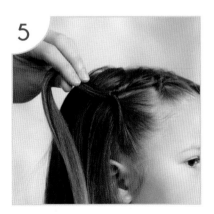

STEP 5 Make a second ponytail with this section of hair and be sure to include the hair from the first ponytail. Flip the second ponytail under as shown previously.

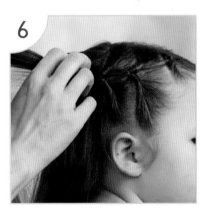

STEP 6 With the remaining hair above the ear, make a third ponytail and flip it under as was done before.

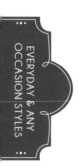

EVERYDAY & ANY OCCASION STYLES

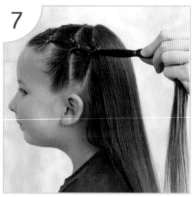

STEP 7 Repeat steps 2–7 on the left side of the head so there are 3 flipped ponytails. Be sure the parts line up that run across the head. Then about 2 inches behind the last ponytail on the left, wrap another elastic around the hair.

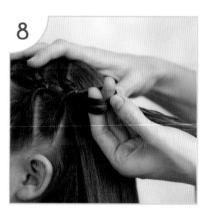

STEP 8 With your fingers, make a hole through the hair in front of the elastic you just added in step 7.

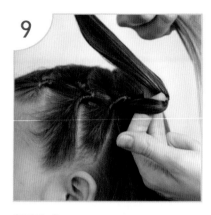

STEP 9 Flip the end of the ponytail up and, with your fingers that are coming through the hole, pull the ends of the ponytail through.

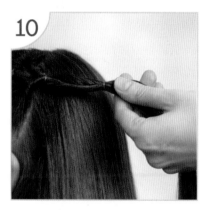

STEP 10 This flips the ponytail and creates the look of a fishbone braid.

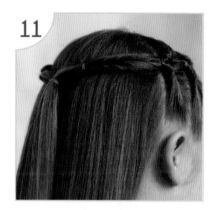

STEP 11 On the right side ponytail, add another elastic 2 inches behind the last ponytail. Repeat steps 9–10 to create another fake fishbone braided section. Then, with an elastic join the ends of the ponytails together in the middle of the head.

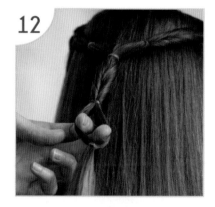

STEP 12 Below the elastic in the middle, add another elastic a few inches below and as done in previous steps, flip the ponytail through. Repeat this process as many times as desired down the ponytail.

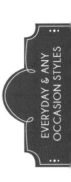

13

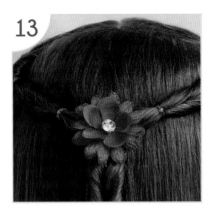

STEP 13 If desired, add a cute little flower or accessory in the middle where the ponytails join. Mist entire hairstyle with hair spray.

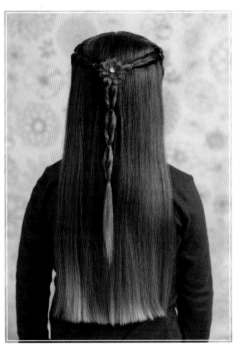

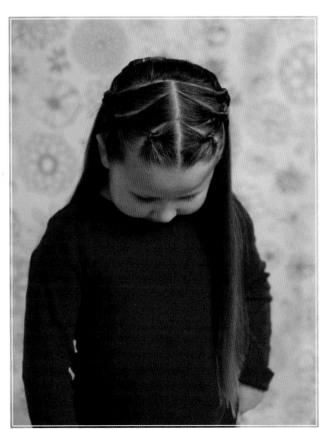

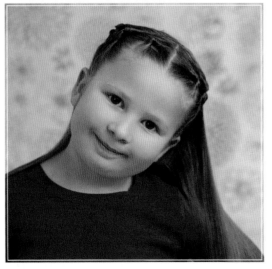

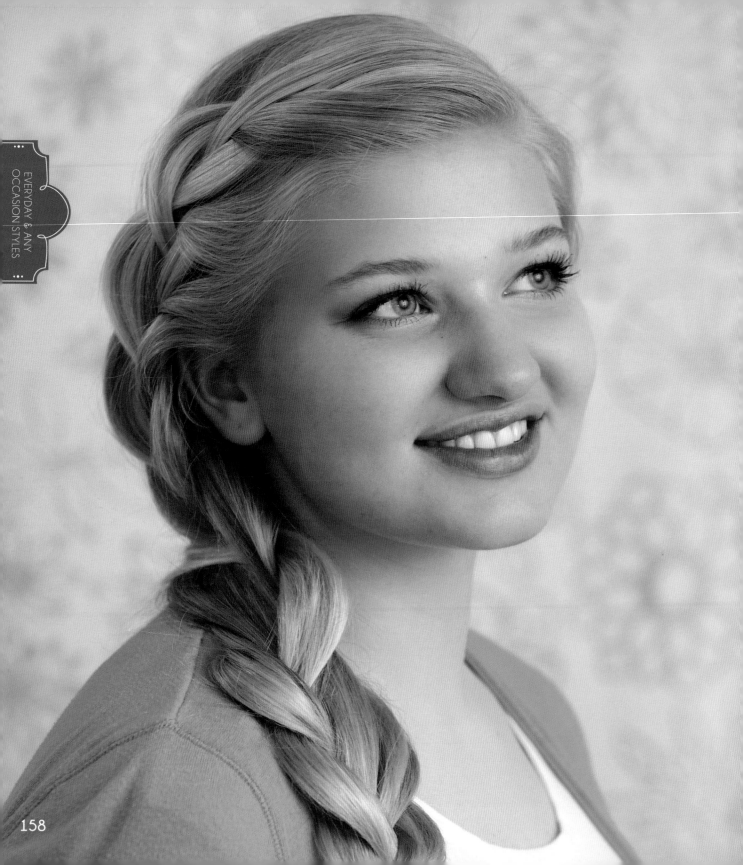

PANCAKED SIDESWEPT FRENCH BRAID

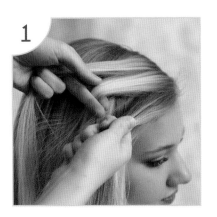

1

STEP 1 Make a part on the left side of the head back to the crown (or on the right side if preferred.) Grasp a section of hair along the hairline above the forehead and divide it into 3 sections.

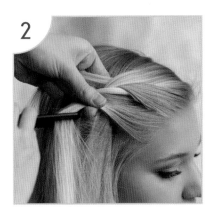

2

STEP 2 Begin making a lace braid (one-sided French braid) as shown on page 26, except add hair from the right side near the face. When adding hair to the braid, make sure they are thick sections.

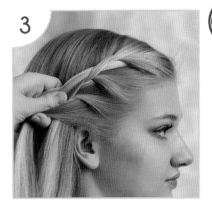

3

STEP 3 Continue braiding only adding hair to the right side until you reach the ear. Since you want a looser thicker look to the braid, you should only have had to add hair 3–4 times to the braid. Before step 4, be sure to cross the left section of the braid over to become the middle section because you will add to it.

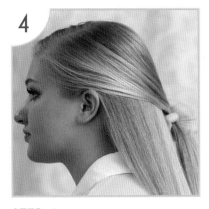

4

STEP 4 From the left side, grab hair along the hairline and left ear and draw it across the back of the head to the braid on the right.

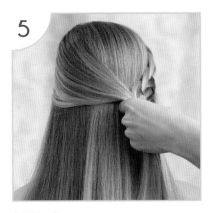

5

STEP 5 Add this hair into the section that is now in the middle of the braid from step 3.

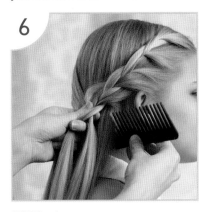

6

STEP 6 Cross the section on the right side of the braid over to the middle position and with your comb, add more hair to it. Then cross the section of hair on the left over to become the middle position of the braid.

159

EVERYDAY & ANY OCCASION STYLES

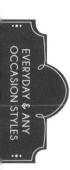

7

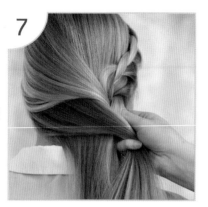

8

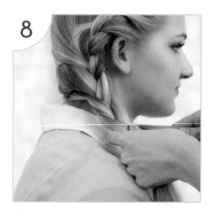

9

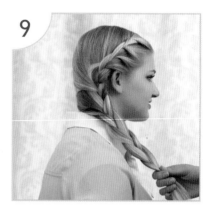

STEP 7 Grab more hair from the left side of the head and draw it over to the braid. Add it to the section that is currently the middle section of the braid from the end of step 6. Cross the right section of the braid over to the middle, but do not add any hair to it.

STEP 8 Gather the remaining hair from the neckline on the left side and incorporate it into the French braid. There should be no more hair to add into the braid after this.

STEP 9 Continue plaiting a regular 3-strand braid until you reach the end of the hair.

10

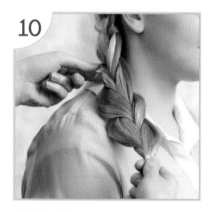

11

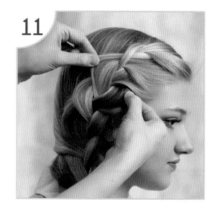

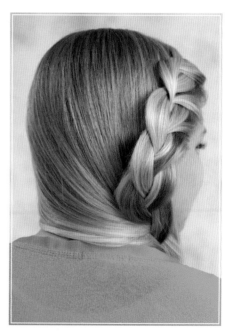

STEP 10 While loosely holding the end of the braid with one hand, start tugging on the edges of the braid with the other to pancake it and make it wider. Once the bottom of the braid is wide as you like, secure the end with an elastic.

STEP 11 Carefully pull on the edges of the braid along the face to pancake them as well. Once desired look is achieved, mist with finishing spray.

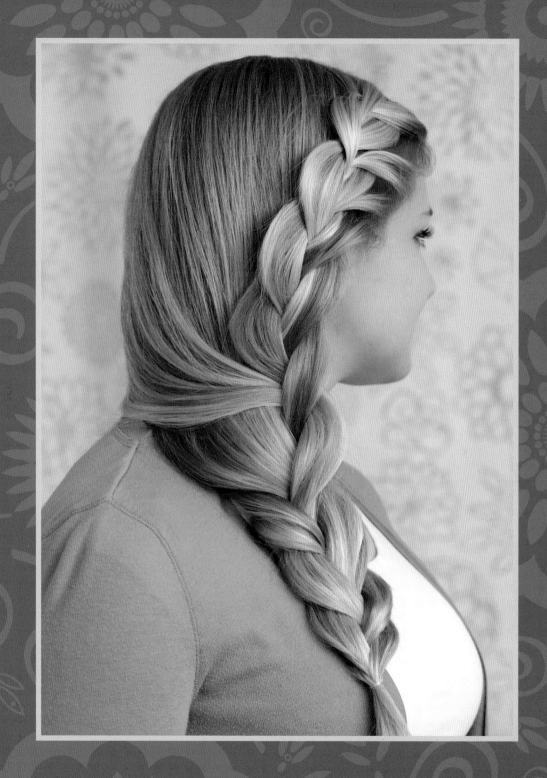

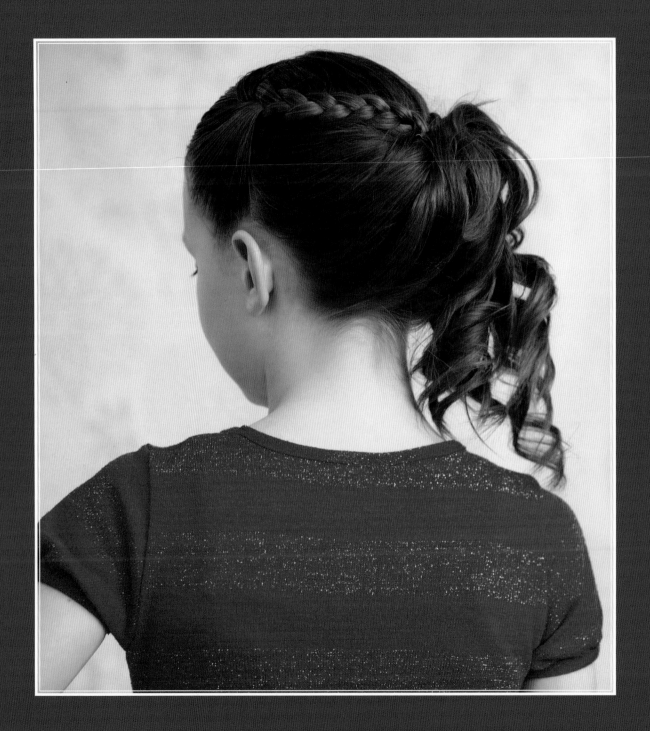

CHAPTER 5

Elegant Updos & Special Occasion Styles

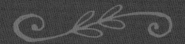

Elegant Updos & Special Occasion Styles

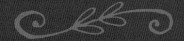

Whether you're going out for a night on the town, heading to prom, or just wanting to look extra nice for church, all eyes will be on you!

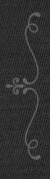

PRETTY UPDOS and elegant styles are my all-time favorite hairstyles to create! Are you heading out for a night on the town, going to a formal dance, attending a wedding, or want to look extra nice for church? These styles are perfect for those extra special occasions when looking your best is a must!

Some of these styles are obviously more advanced and definitely more time consuming. If you aren't as skilled at doing hair, you might find it helpful to have a friend around to lend a hand. If it is an extra special occasion, I also recommend practicing the hairstyle days before the actual event to know how long it will take and how it will turn out.

As with all the other styles, you are being an artist and creating something beautiful. Have fun exploring other ways of achieving new and beautiful hairstyles.

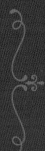

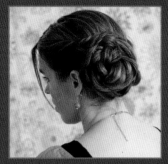

BRAIDED UPDO
167

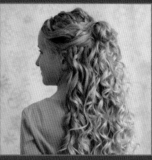

CASCADING CURLS
171

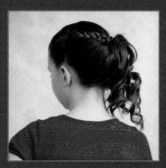

SWEPT UP CURLS
& BRAIDS
175

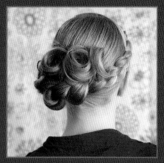

DUTCH BRAID &
CURLS UPDO
179

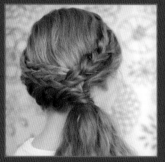

BOHO BRAIDS & TWIST
183

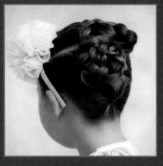

OFFSET DOUBLE BUNS
187

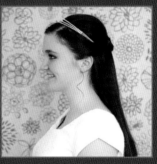

HALF-UP LOOPS
& TWISTS
191

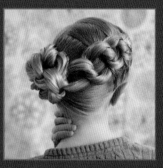

KNOTTED UPDO
195

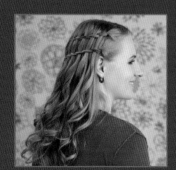

DOUBLE
WATERFALL TWIST
199

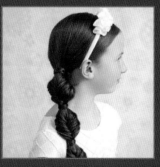

FISHBONE BUBBLES
203

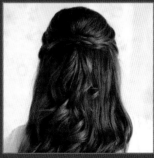

BRAIDED PULLBACK
& CURLS
207

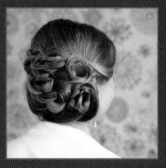

4-STRAND BRAID UPDO
211

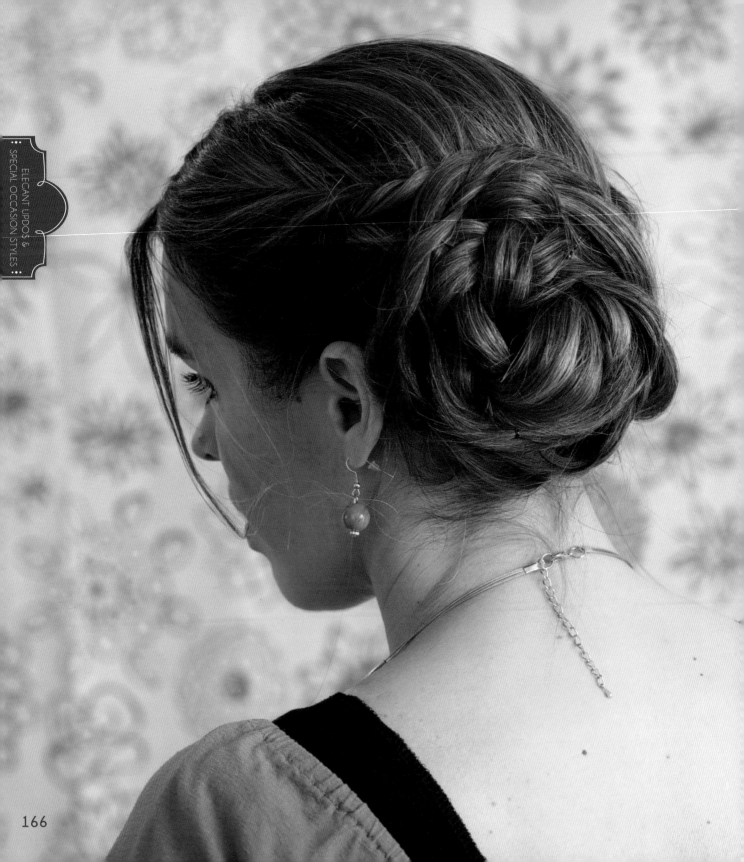

BRAIDED UPDO

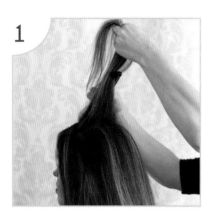

STEP 1 At the crown, backcomb hair to add a bit of volume. Flip the hair back down that has been back-combed and with a comb, gently smooth the top layer of hair.

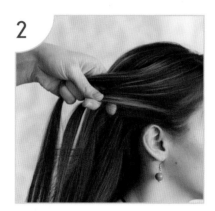

STEP 2 On the right side of the head, above the ear, section out a piece of hair and divide it into three sec-tions. Braid one rotation of a regular 3-strand braid (right piece over middle piece, left piece over middle piece.)

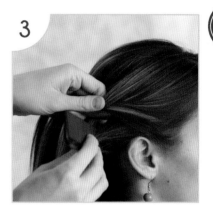

STEP 3 Only add hair to the right (or bottom) section of hair and begin to make a lace braid a.k.a. one-sided French braid (see page 26).

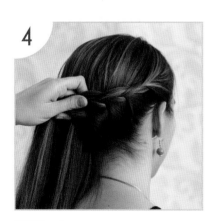

STEP 4 Continue the lace braid around the head, only adding hair to the bottom section of hair. Be careful to keep the hair smooth on the back of the head.

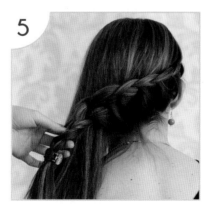

STEP 5 Once the left side of the neck is reached, stop adding hair and make a regular 3-strand braid down the section of hair. Secure the braid temporarily with a claw clip.

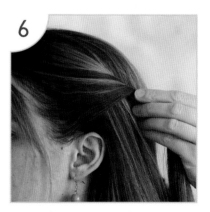

STEP 6 Move to the left side of the head and section out a small piece of hair in front of the ear.

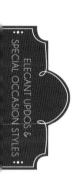

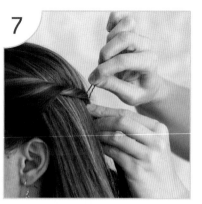

STEP 7 Twist the section of hair several times. Pull the twisted hair back and secure with a bobby pin to the hair in back.

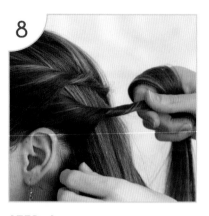

STEP 8 Take a second section of hair from behind the ear below the first twist. Twist this section of hair several times.

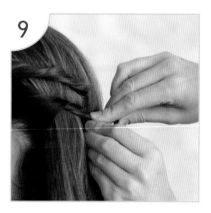

STEP 9 Secure the second twist with a bobby pin just below the first twist. There will still be straight hair hanging down on the left side that you will work with in later steps.

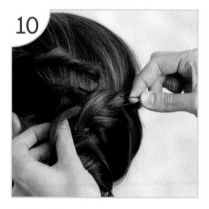

STEP 10 Draw the edge of the lace braid upward until it touches the bottom twist. Secure with bobby pins as needed.

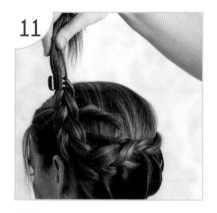

STEP 11 Draw the remaining part of the braid up and around in a clockwise direction to begin wrapping a loose bun.

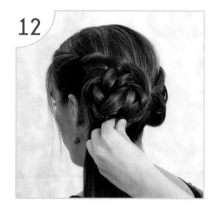

STEP 12 Remove the claw clip and secure the bun with bobby pins. Carefully tuck the tail of the braid around and under the bun as you are able. Secure with bobby pins as needed.

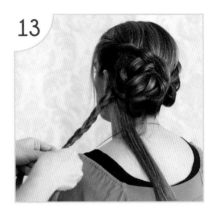

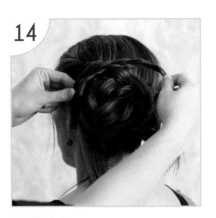

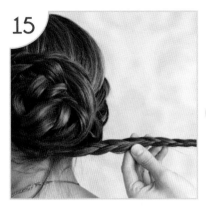

STEP 13 With the remaining straight hair, divide it into two sections. Make a regular 3-strand braid with the section on the left.

STEP 14 Draw the small braid up and around the left side and over the top of the bun. Tuck the ends in to hide them and secure with bobby pins.

STEP 15 With the remaining hair, make another 3-strand braid.

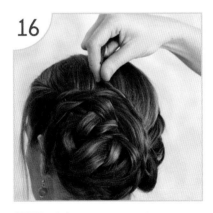

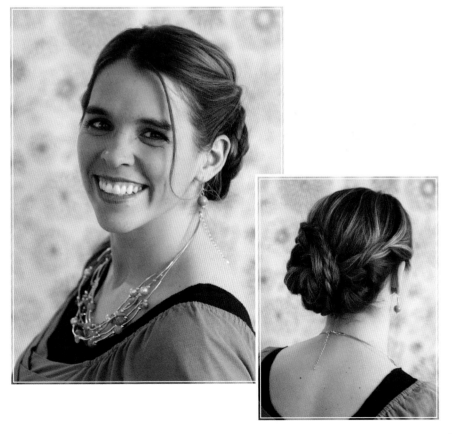

STEP 16 Draw the braid up and around the right side of the bun. Tuck the ends in to hide them and secure with bobby pins. Smooth and tuck in any stray hairs as needed and spray with finishing spray.

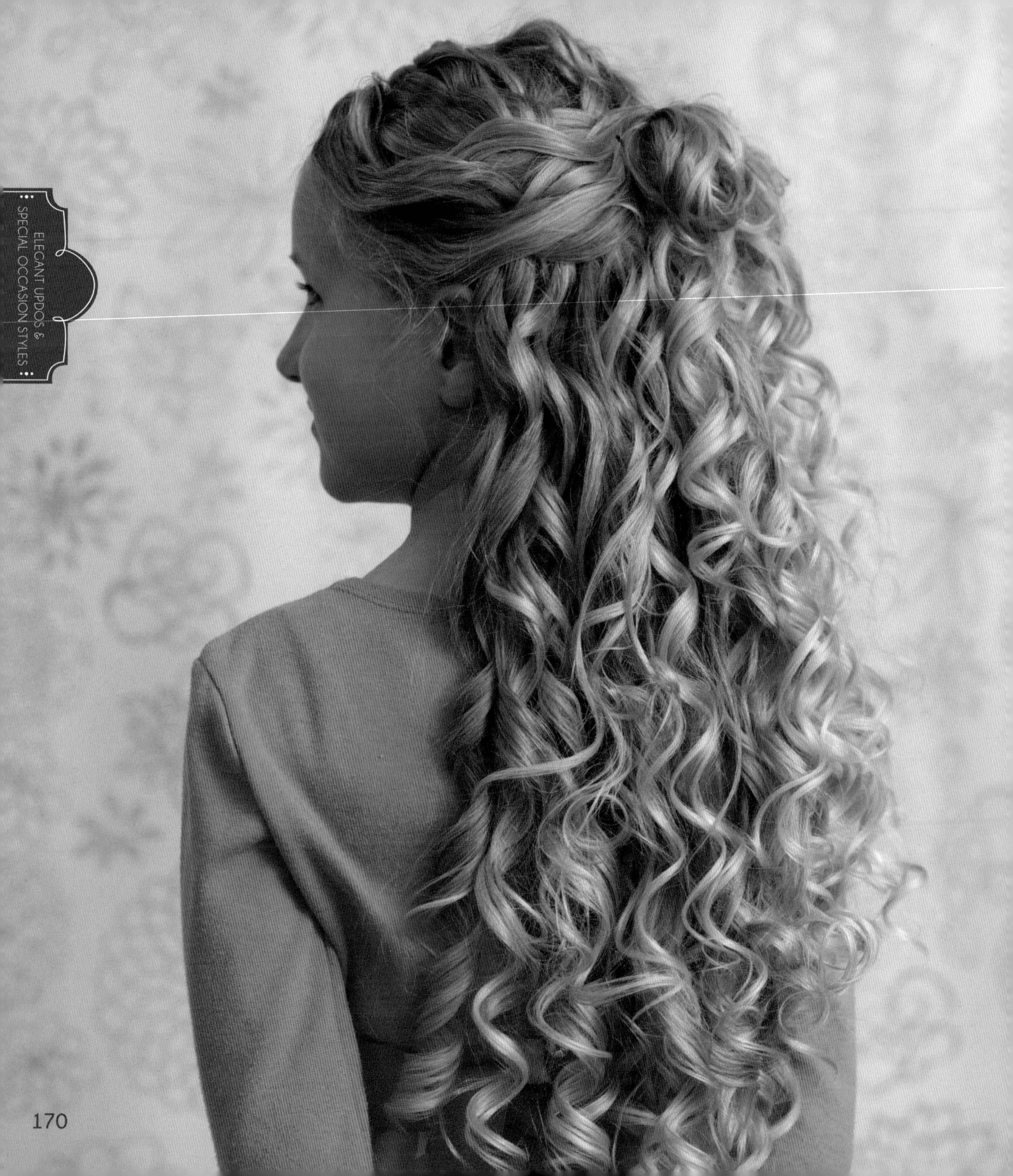

CASCADING CURLS

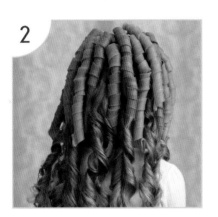

STEP 1 Wash hair and massage mouse throughout wet hair. Set entire head of hair in favorite curlers. If rollers or curlers are not available, curl all your hair with a curling iron or wand.

STEP 2 Allow the hair to completely dry before removing curlers. Starting at the nape of the neck, work your way up through the hair and remove the curlers.

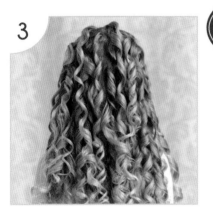

STEP 3 Once all the curlers have been removed, apply an anti-frizz serum if needed.

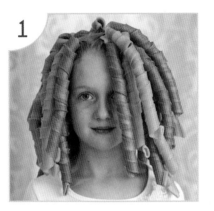

STEP 4 Divide each curl into 3–4 sections to add volume to the curls and to break up any ringlets

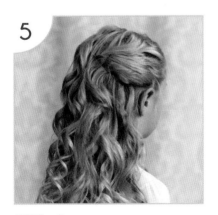

STEP 5 On the right side near the ear, gently comb the curls back with your fingers. Secure the hair by making an X with a couple bobby pins on the side of the head.

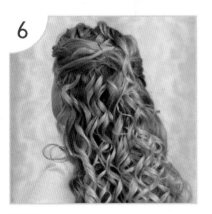

STEP 6 Repeat on the left side of the head and secure with bobby pins.

171

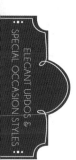

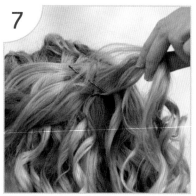

STEP 7 Take a section of curls from the right of the bobby pins in Step 6.

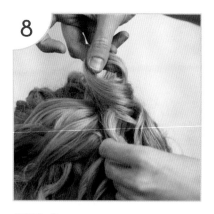

STEP 8 Draw the curls upward and twist them once to form a loop.

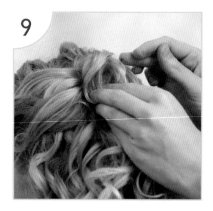

STEP 9 Place the loop of curls over the X of bobby pins from Step 6 and secure with a bobby pin.

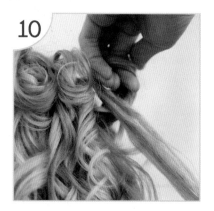

STEP 10 Repeat the process of taking a section of curl from the back of the head, making a loop and securing it with a bobby pin. There should be 3–4 of these curled loops across the back of the head and the bobby pin X's from step 5 and 6 should be covered with these loops.

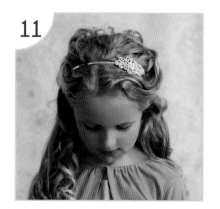

STEP 11 Add a pretty tiara or headband to dress the style up even more. Arrange any other curls that need to be adjusted. Mist with finishing spray.

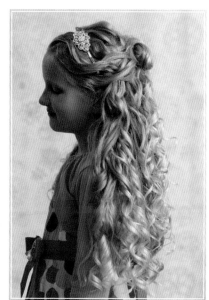

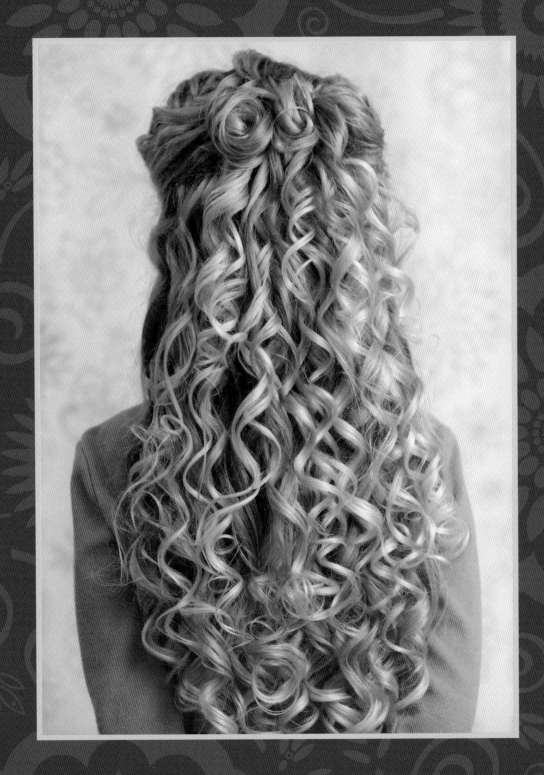

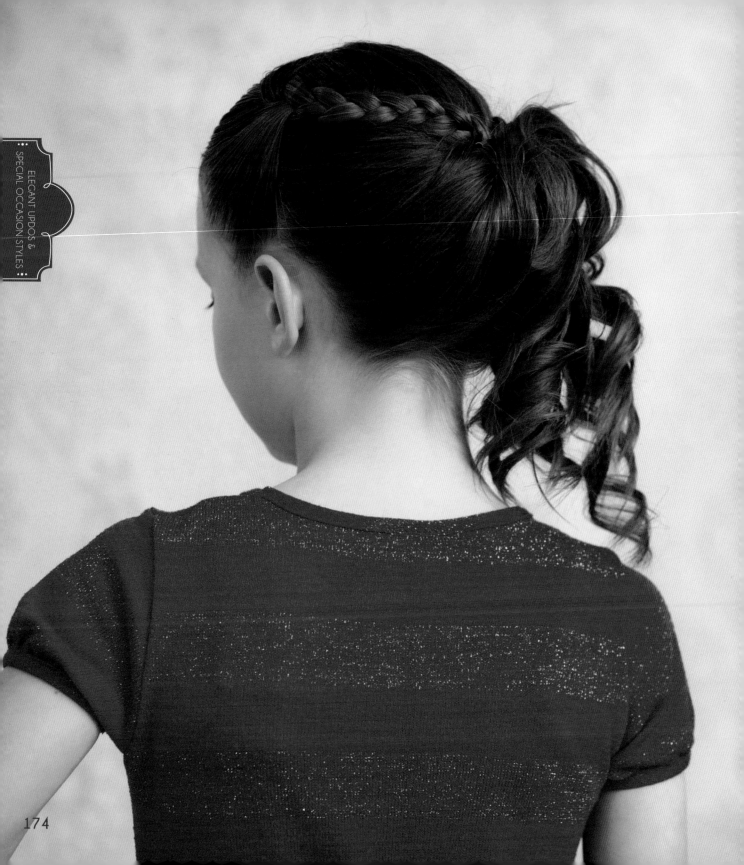

SWEPT-UP CURLS & BRAIDS

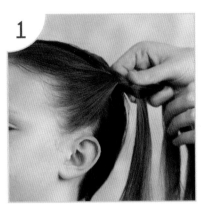

STEP 1 Make a side part on the right side of the head back to the crown. Make another part branching off it down to the left ear. Begin a regular 3-strand braid as shown on page 22.

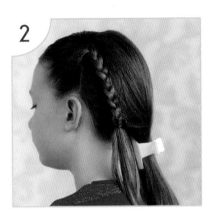

STEP 2 Braid far enough down until the braid can reach around the back of the head to the right side. Temporarily secure the end with a small claw clip.

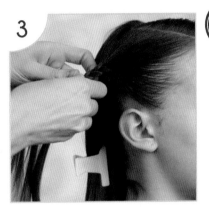

STEP 3 On the right side, repeat the above steps parting down to the ear and plait a regular 3-strand braid.

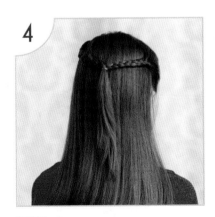

STEP 4 Bring the 2 braids together in the back and join them with a hair elastic. Remove the small clip from step 2. Position the elastic toward the right side of the head.

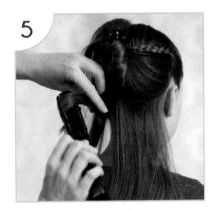

STEP 5 Divide the remaining hair in back in half. Clip the top half out of the way and curl the bottom layer.

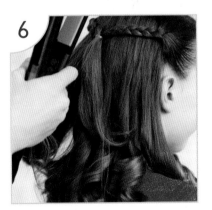

STEP 6 Once the bottom layer is curled, release the clip and let the remaining hair down. Curl the rest of the straight hair.

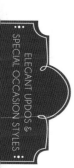

7

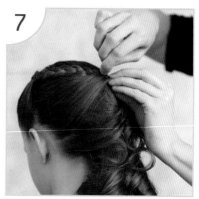

8

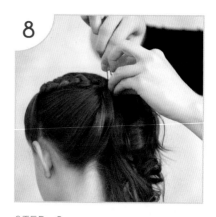

9

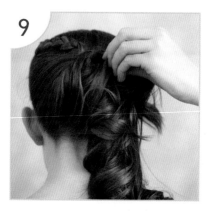

STEP 7 On the left side, gently draw a large section of hair from the neck up toward the braids. Slightly twist the hair inward and secure it with bobby pins to cover up the elastic from step 4.

STEP 8 Take any remaining hair on the left side and draw it upward toward the braid and secure it with a bobby pin.

STEP 9 Draw a third section of hair upward from the middle of the neck and secure with a bobby pin next to the one in step 8.

10

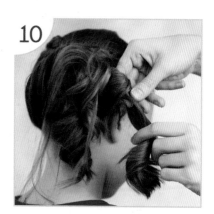

STEP 10 On the right side of the head, take a curled section and draw it upward toward the braid on the right. Secure as needed with bobby pins. Pin up any remaining loose pieces of hair and re-curl sections if needed. Gently run your fingers through the curls a bit to break them up if desired. Spray completed style with holding spray.

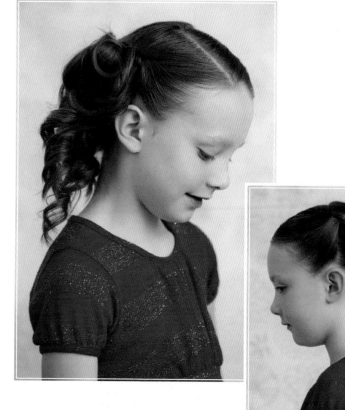

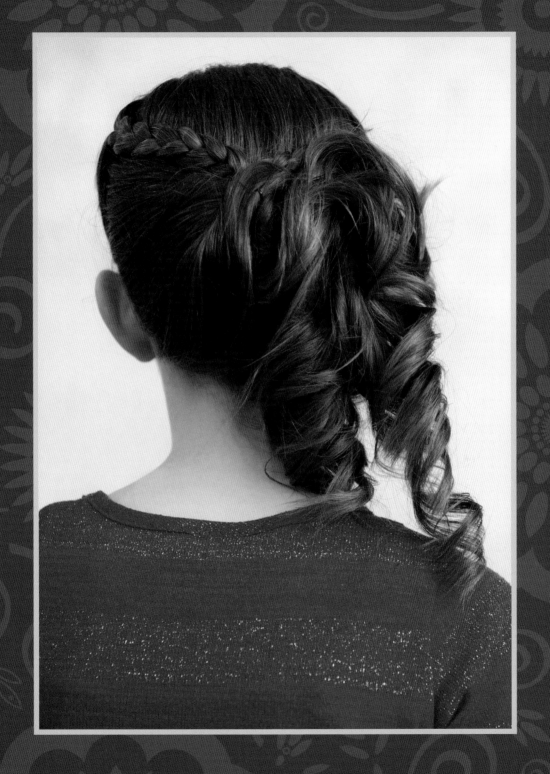

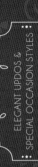

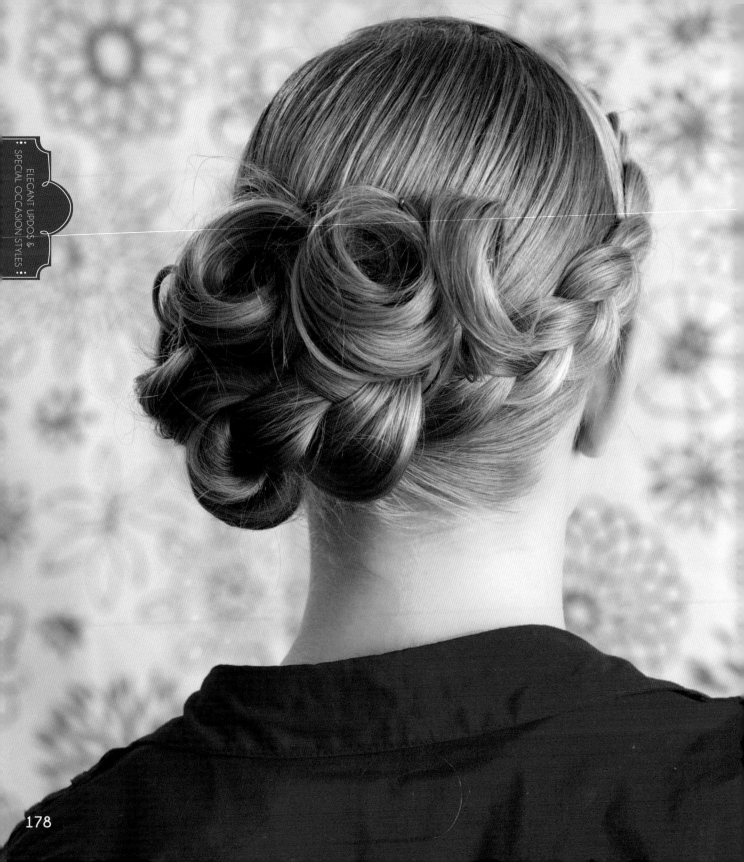

DUTCH BRAID & CURLS UPDO

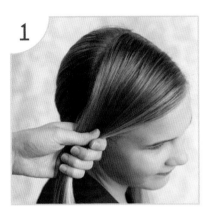

STEP 1 Part the hair on the left side of the head back to the crown, and then down to the right ear.

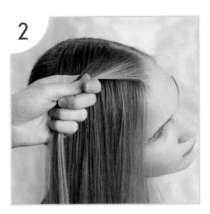

STEP 2 Part out a small triangular section of hair along the hairline.

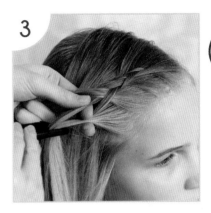

STEP 3 Begin making a Dutch French braid. This is made just like a regular French braid as shown on page 28, but instead of crossing the strands of hair over each other, you pass the hair under. This type of braid can also be called an inside-out French braid because it sits on top of the head and is more 3D. A Dutch French braid is optional and if you prefer, create a regular French braid.

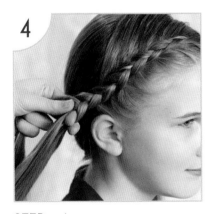

STEP 4 Once you reach the right ear, stop adding hair into the braid and continue making a regular 3-strand braid halfway down the hair. Secure the end of the braid temporarily with a clip.

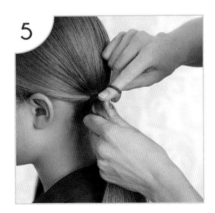

STEP 5 Gather all the remaining hair into a low ponytail behind the left ear and secure with a ponytail holder.

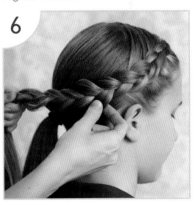

STEP 6 Remove the clip from the braid. Start at the end of the braid and begin to pancake the braid by gently tugging on the sides of the braid to make it wider and flatter (as shown on page 23).

179

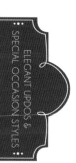

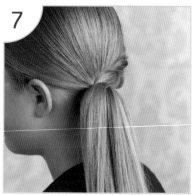

STEP 7 Once the braid is to your liking, secure the braid to the ponytail with a clear elastic.

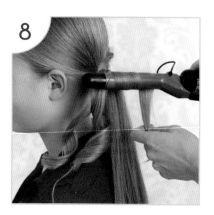

STEP 8 With a 1" curling iron, take small sections of hair from the top of the ponytail and proceed to curl 4–5 pieces. Mist them with hair spray after curling each one.

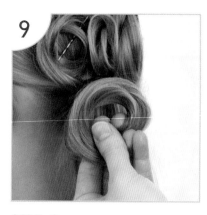

STEP 9 Take each individual curl, wrap it around your fingers in a circular fashion, and gently ease it off so it makes a circle of hair, or a pin curl.

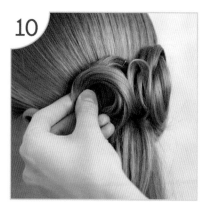

STEP 10 With bobby pins, secure as needed to the hair just above the base of the ponytail. You should have 4 or 5 pin curls when you are done. For added dimension secure the first 3 pin curls right to the head and then the last couple on top of those. Mist with hair spray to ensure they hold their shape.

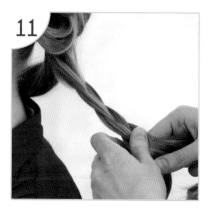

STEP 11 Loosely curl the remaining hair of the ponytail and then divide it in half. With the left section make a loose regular 3-strand braid. Don't braid all the way to the end. You will use the curly ends in a later step.

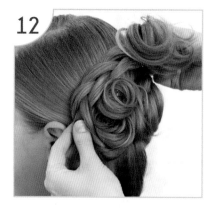

STEP 12 Draw the braid up and around the left side of the pin curls and secure with bobby pins as needed so the braid doesn't unravel. For now, leave the curly ends free to fall over the top of the pin curls.

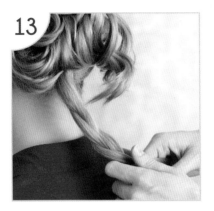

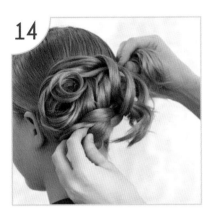

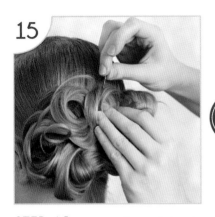

STEP 13 Take the last of the pony-tail and make another loose 3-strand braid.

STEP 14 Position the braid under the pin curls at the base of the hair-style. Draw the curled ends up and around the pin curls to the right side. Secure the braid with bobby pins but leave the curled ends of the braid free.

STEP 15 Arrange the curled ends of each braid as desired so they form similar circles or pin curls and secure with bobby pins or hair pins. Mist entire style with hair spray.

ELEGANT UPDOS & SPECIAL OCCASION STYLES

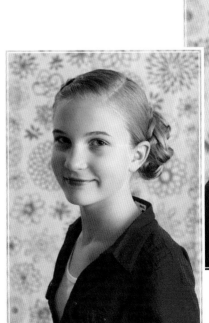

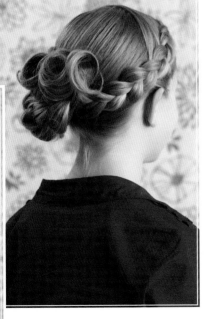

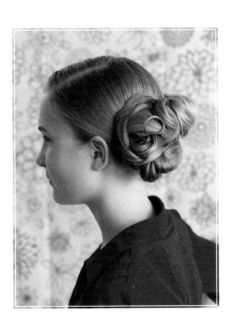

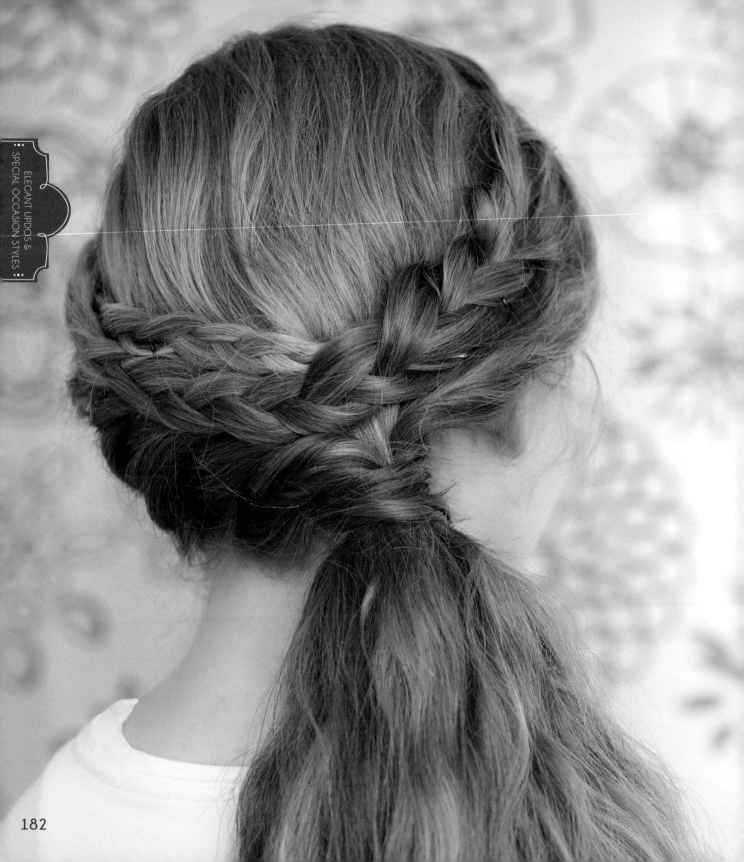

The beauty of updos is there are endless ways to create them. The downfall to that is there isn't always exactness to them. Based on your preference, the style may change if you chose to create a different braid or secure the curls in different places.

BOHO BRAIDS & TWIST

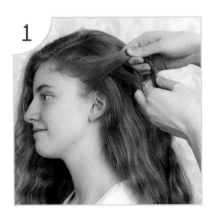

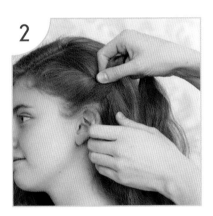

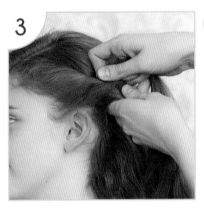

STEP 1 Make a side part on the left side of the head. At the hairline, take a small section of hair in front of the left ear and divide it into two pieces. Cross the bottom piece over the top piece of hair so they trade places and make an X.

STEP 2 Let the section that is now in the bottom position drop and hang down with the rest of the hair. Add a small section of hair from the hairline near the ear, to the piece of hair you just dropped (as done in French Rope Twists on page 137).

STEP 3 Take that entire section of hair and pass it over the top piece so they trade places. Now let section of hair that is on bottom drop and hang down with the rest of the hair. Grab hair from below, along with the piece of hair you just dropped.

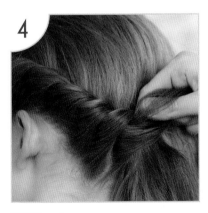

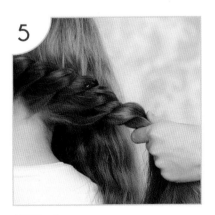

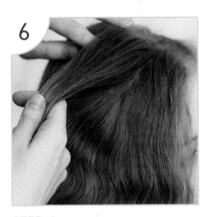

STEP 4 Continue the process around the hairline, adding hair to the bottom section you drop and then cross it over to the top position.

STEP 5 Repeat the process of the twist until you reach the right side of the neck. Be sure to keep the twist at the base of the neck. Stop adding hair and twist the hair a few times and temporarily secure the twist with a clip.

STEP 6 On the right side of the head grasp a 1 1/2-inch section of hair, leaving hair out in front along the face.

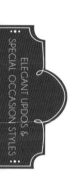

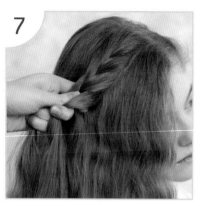

STEP 7 Proceed to make a French Braid as shown on page 28, but make it fairly loose and take chunky sections.

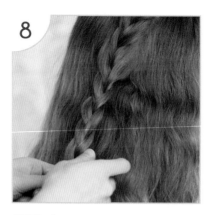

STEP 8 Once you reach the top of the right ear, stop adding hair into the French braid and continue braiding a regular 3-strand braid until you reach the end of the hair. Secure with an elastic.

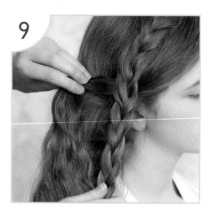

STEP 9 Draw the remaining hair in front of the French braid back toward the right ear. Bring the hair underneath the braid.

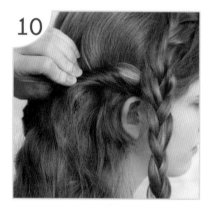

STEP 10 Gently twist the hair toward the head and secure with a few bobby pins

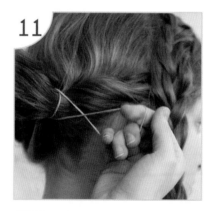

STEP 11 Combine all the hair except the braid into a low side ponytail behind the right ear and secure with a ponytail holder.

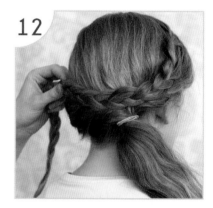

STEP 12 Drape the braid across the back of the head so it rests just above the twisted hair from the beginning steps of the hairstyle.

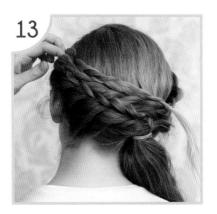

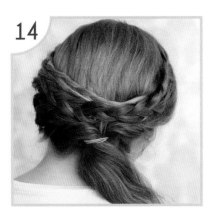

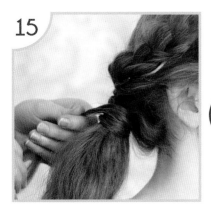

STEP 13 Secure the braid as needed with bobby pins. Once the braid reaches where the twist starts on the left side, if you have enough hair, fold the braid and bring it back in the opposite direction. If you are working with shorter hair, simply tuck the tail of the braid under and secure with bobby pins.

STEP 14 Tuck the tail and elastic of the braid in to hide it and secure with bobby pins as needed.

STEP 15 Cover the ponytail holder with hair as shown on page 36.

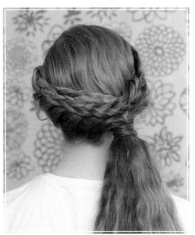

QUICK TIP

TO ACHIEVE A MORE "bohemian-like" look, loosely braid your hair the night before. This will create flowing waves the next day that will add so much more to the style than having straight hair.

BONUS STYLE

SKIP STEPS 1–5 and make a gorgeous wrapped braid instead.

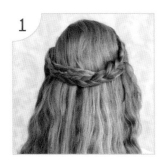

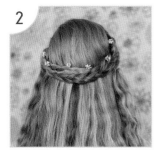

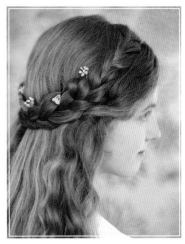

STEP 1 Start with step 6 from previous page and create a braid. Omit making a ponytail and drape the braid as shown in Steps 12–14

STEP 2 Add a few small flowers to add to the bohemian look.

185

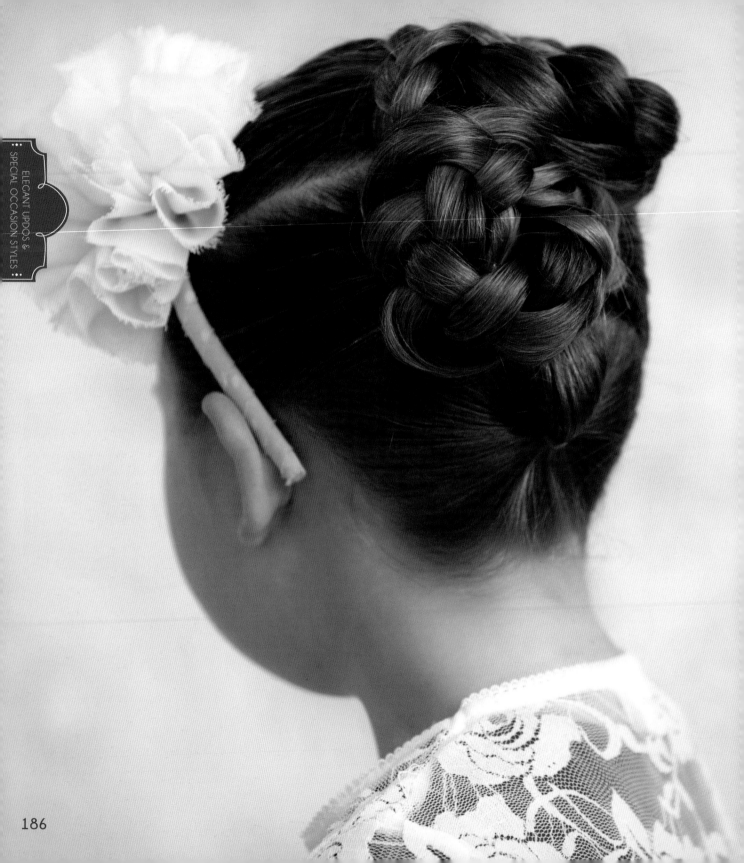

OFFSET DOUBLE BUNS

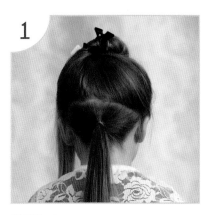

STEP 1 Part the hair around the back of the head from ear to ear. Clip all the hair from above up out of the way. Make a low ponytail in back with the remaining hair.

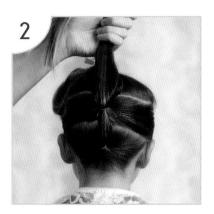

STEP 2 Next, part around the back of the head from temple to temple. Gather that section of hair into a ponytail and include the ponytail from step 1. Secure just above the first ponytail with another elastic.

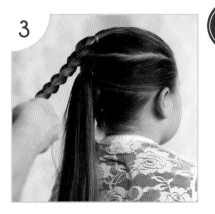

STEP 3 With the remaining hair on top, create a third ponytail at the center of the crown and secure with an elastic. Do not include the ponytail from step 2. Make a regular 3-strand braid as shown on page 22. Secure the end of the braid with an elastic.

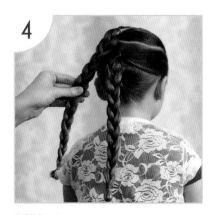

STEP 4 Plait a braid in the ponytail from step 2 and secure the end with an elastic.

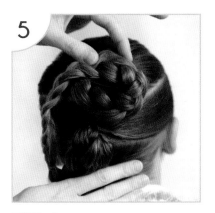

STEP 5 Draw the top braid to the right and in a counterclockwise direction wrap the braid. Don't create a tight bun. Secure the braid with bobby pins so it forms a sideways oval.

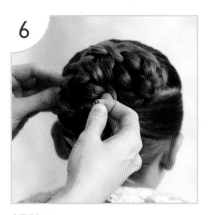

STEP 6 Draw the bottom braid to the left of the top bun. Wrap it in a clockwise direction. Secure with bobby pins as needed so it is not directly under the top bun. Position it so it allows the ponytail from Step 1 to show.

187

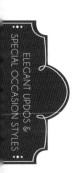

7

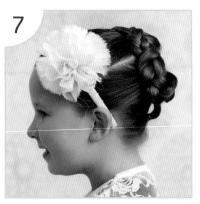

STEP 7 Add a fun headband or other accessory if desired.

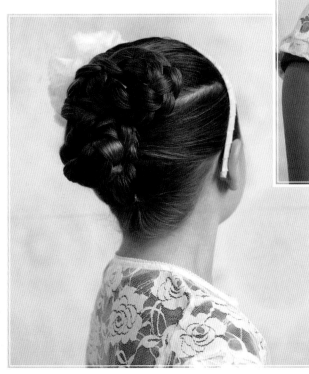

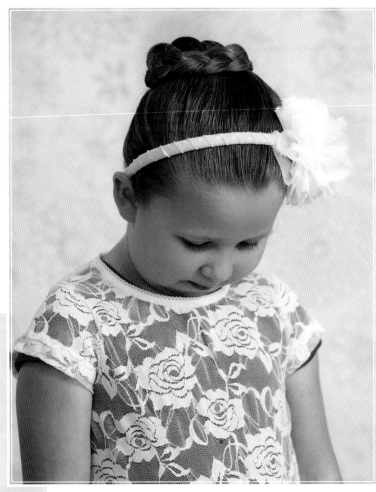

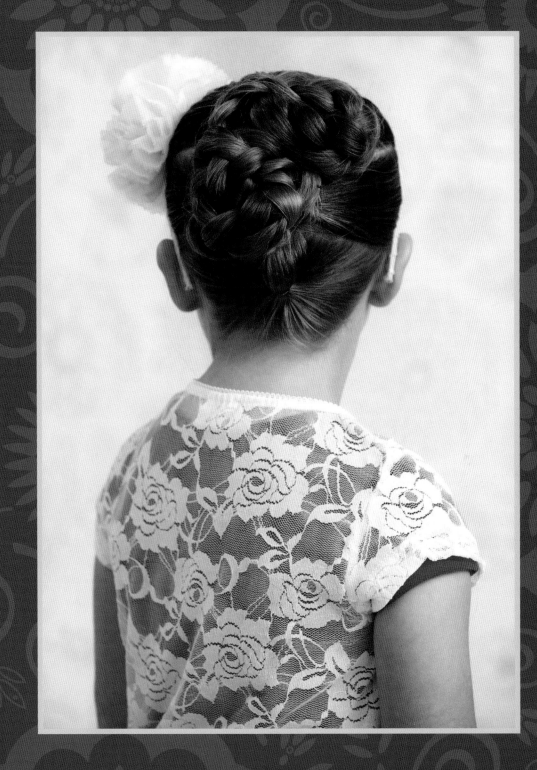

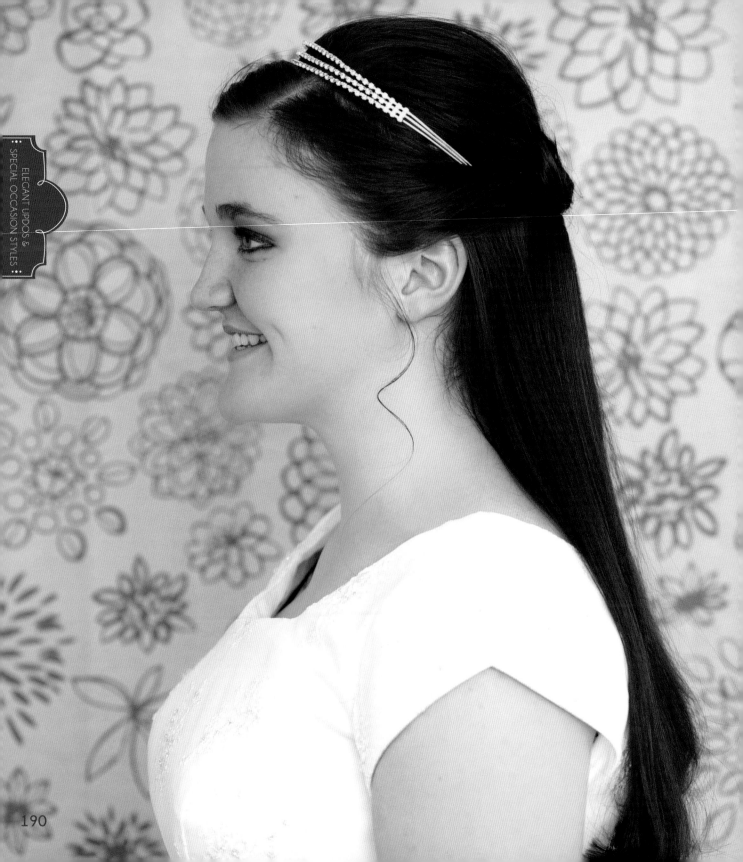

HALF-UP LOOPS & TWISTS

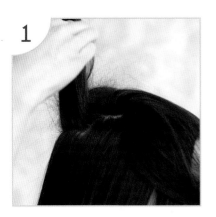

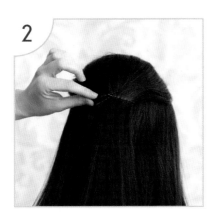

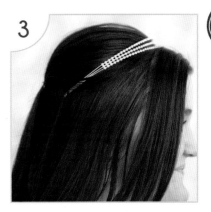

STEP 1 Starting at the crown, backcomb the hair to add volume. Backcomb several sections and mist the underside of each section with hair spray for a better hold. For a bigger bouffant or poof, back comb more hair.

STEP 2 Flip the hair back and smooth out the top layer of hair. Draw the hair back at each temple to make a slight bouffant or poof. Secure it in back with a couple of bobby pins. Don't pull all the hair back that is above the ears at this time.

STEP 3 Be sure to leave out several inches of hair in front along the face. Add a headband or tiara at an angle as shown in the picture.

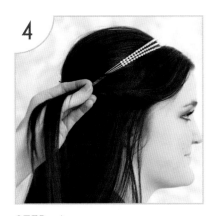

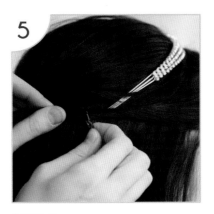

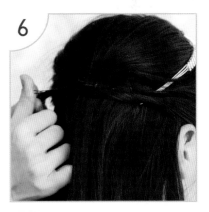

STEP 4 On the right side of the head, take a small section of hair in front of the headband and twist in toward the head.

STEP 5 Draw the twisted hair backward and anchor it with a bobby pin to the right of the bobby pins in Step 3. If possible, try to cover the end of the headband as well.

STEP 6 With the remaining hair by the right ear, twist it toward the head and draw it around the back of the head. Bring the twisted hair over the bobby pins from Step 3. Secure the twist with a bobby pin on the left of all the bobby pins.

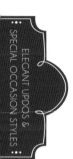

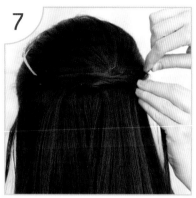

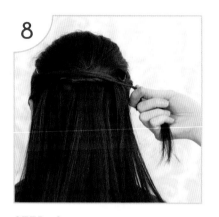

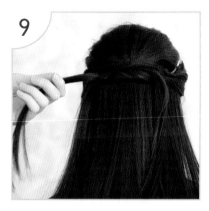

STEP 7 On the left side of the head, repeat what was done on the right side. Take half the hair that is near the face and twist it in toward the head. Draw it to the right side of the head and anchor it near the bobby pin from step 5.

STEP 8 With the remaining hair above the left ear, repeat the process and twist the hair in toward the head and drape it across the back on the other twists. Secure on the far right side with another bobby pin.

STEP 9 Mist the "tail" from the twist in Step 6 with hair spray or other product to make the hair easier to form pin curls.

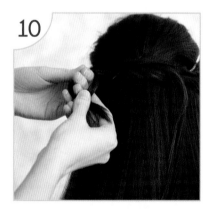

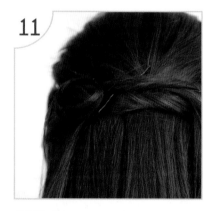

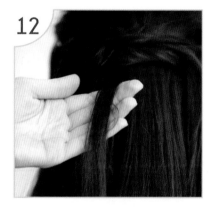

STEP 10 Wrap this hair around your fingers to form a circle of hair.

STEP 11 Gently ease it off your fingers and place it on top of the twists. Secure with bobby pins to the left side of the bouffant.

STEP 12 From the center back of the head, take a small piece of hair and repeat the process, misting it with hair spray.

13

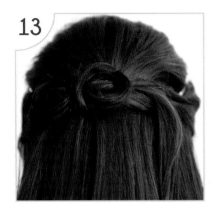

STEP 13 Draw this hair upward, wrapping it around your fingers as shown in the previous steps. Place the coiled hair to the right of the one in Step 12. Secure it with bobby pins or hair pins as needed.

14A

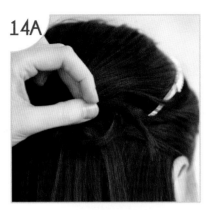

14B

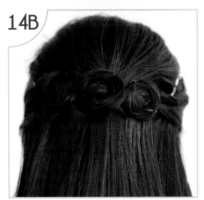

STEPS 14A & 14B Repeat the process a third time using the tail of the twist from Step 7 to create the pin curl. Secure with bobby pins or hair pins to the right of the middle pin curl.

15

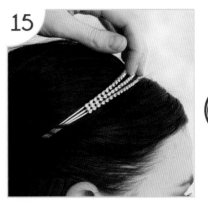

STEP 15 Adjust the headband as needed and if desired, curl the hair down in back.

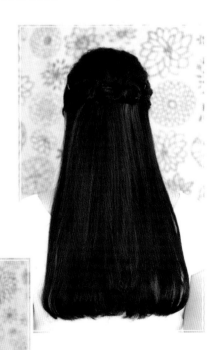

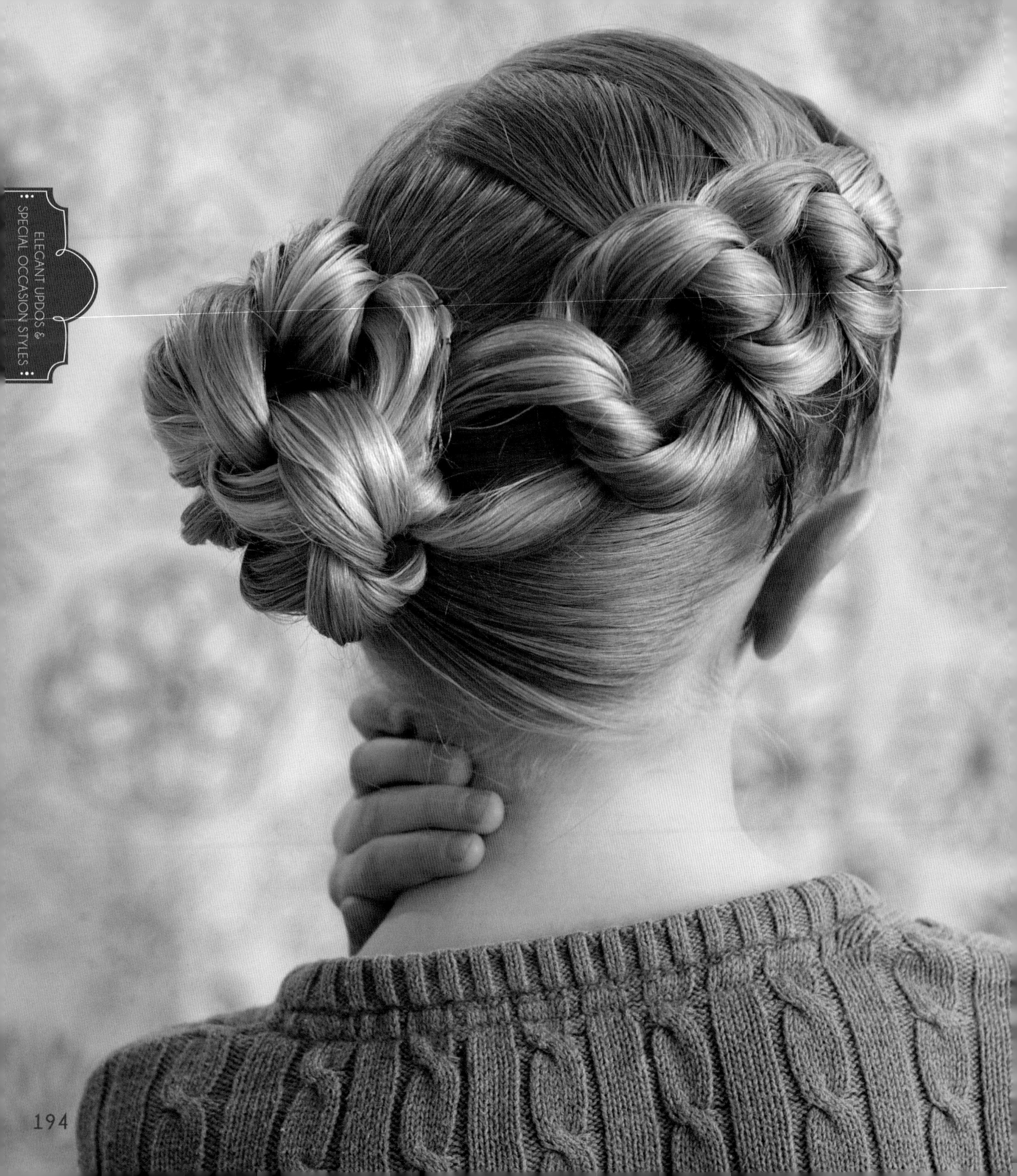

KNOTTED UPDO

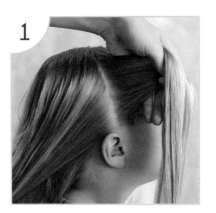

STEP 1 Make a part on the top left side of the head back to the crown. A few inches back from the hairline branch off from the left part and part down to the front of the right ear.

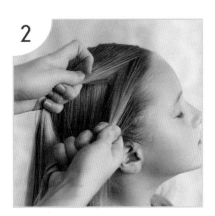

STEP 2 Divide this section of hair into 2 sections.

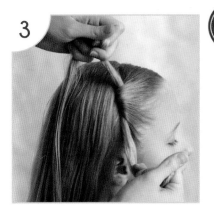

STEP 3 Pass the right section over the left. Then pass it under the left and up through the hole, like when tying your shoe (see page 40). Pull on the ends to bring it tight to the scalp.

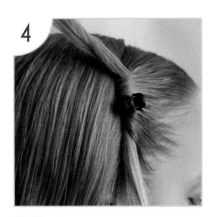

STEP 4 Place a small claw clip around the center of the knot so it does not loosen. Drape the top tail of the knot over the head for now and let the bottom tail hang by the ear.

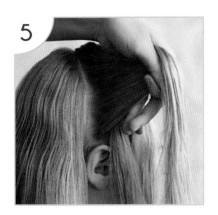

STEP 5 Directly behind the first section, part from the top of the head down to the tip of the right ear.

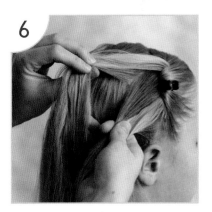

STEP 6 Divide this section in half. Add the left tail of the knot into the left section and the right tail of the knot into the right section.

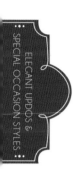

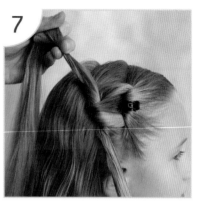

STEP 7 Repeat the knotting process, as done in step 3. Pull it tight and place a claw clip over the center of the knot to secure it.

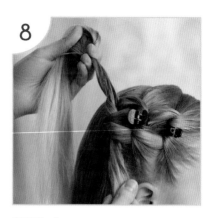

STEP 8 Part out a 3rd section of hair just behind the one in step 5 that goes from the crown down to behind the ear. Repeat the knotting process. Pull it tight and add a claw clip to secure it.

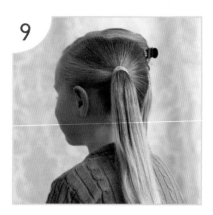

STEP 9 Gather all remaining hair and make a ponytail on the left side of the head. It should sit about level with the of the top of the ear. Secure with a ponytail holder.

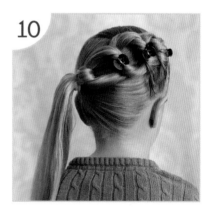

STEP 10 With the remaining hair from the knots, proceed to make two more knots or chains as shown on page 40. You will not be adding hair to these, and do not pull them tight—you want these to be circles. Use claw clips to keep them secured temporarily. Draw these knots back toward the ponytail on the left.

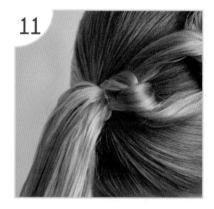

STEP 11 Secure the remaining hair from the knots to the base of the ponytail with an elastic. Carefully remove all the claw clips from the center of the knots.

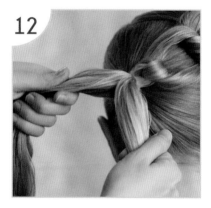

STEP 12 Divide the ponytail into two sections.

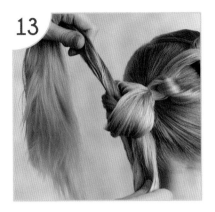

STEP 13 Pass one section over the other and proceed to make a knot, pulling it tight.

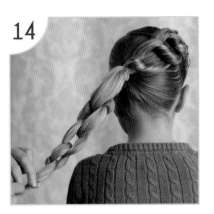

STEP 14 Make knots in the ponytail until you run out of hair. Secure the end with an elastic.

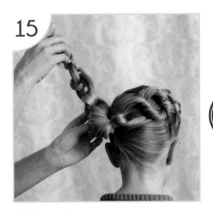

STEP 15 Proceed to wrap the knots in a clockwise direction to form a bun.

ELEGANT UPDOS & SPECIAL OCCASION STYLES

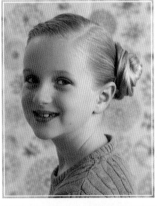

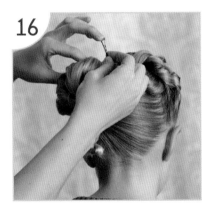

STEP 16 Arrange the bun so it lays nicely and secure with bobby pins as needed.

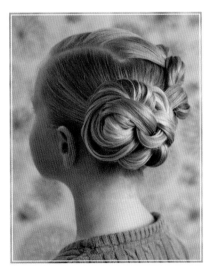

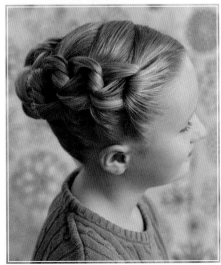

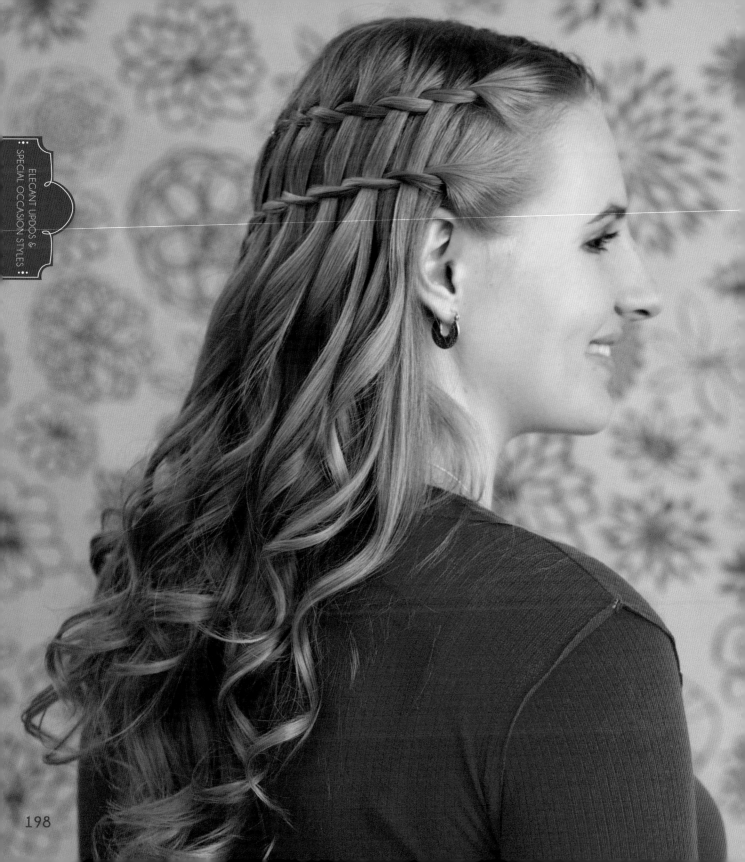

DOUBLE WATERFALL TWIST

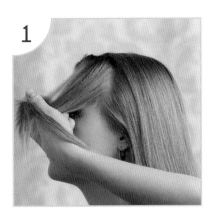

STEP 1 Make a part on the top of the head back to the crown. Starting on the left side of the head, section out a 1 1/2-inch section of hair along the hairline near the left temple.

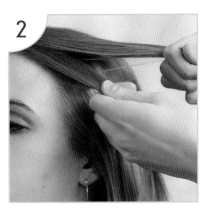

STEP 2 Divide that section of hair into 2 pieces.

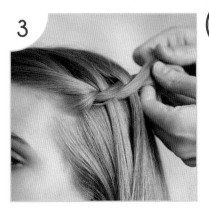

STEP 3 Begin to make a waterfall twist as shown on page 18. Try keeping the twist running straight around the head and not on a diagonal.

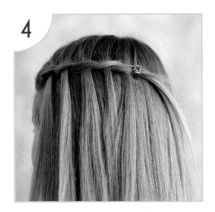

STEP 4 Continue adding sections through the twist until you reach the middle of the back of the head. Temporarily secure the twist to the head with a small claw clip.

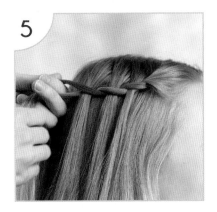

STEP 5 On the right side of the head, starting at the temple, make another waterfall twist.

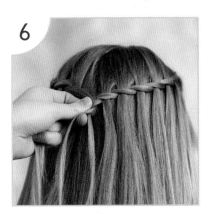

STEP 6 Continue the twist from the right until you reach the middle of the back of the head. Carefully release the clip from the left twist. Join the ends of both twists together in the middle. Secure with a small hair elastic.

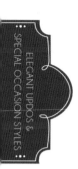

7
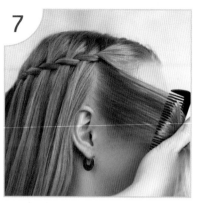

8
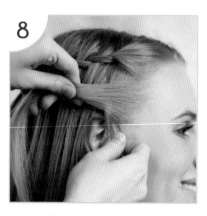

9
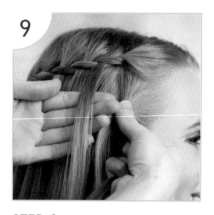

STEP 7 On the right side, just below where you started the twist in step 5, section out the remaining hair in front of the ear.

STEP 8 Divide this section into 2 pieces. Cross the bottom piece over the top to make an X.

STEP 9 For the second layer of this waterfall twist, you will not be adding hair from the hairline. You will use the hair that passed through the twist from the first steps. Grasp the first section of hair that hangs down from the top twist and place it in between the 2 pieces of hair.

10
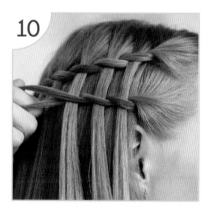

11
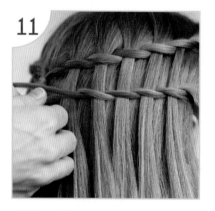

12
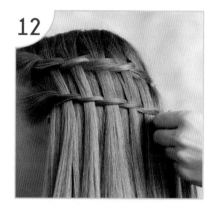

STEP 10 Continue laying the pieces from the first twist in the middle of this new twist. It will create the look of a "ladder" in between the twists.

STEP 11 Keep on twisting and adding hair from the first twist until you reach the elastic from step 6. Temporarily secure the twist with a claw clip.

STEP 12 Repeat steps 7–11 on the left side of the head.

13

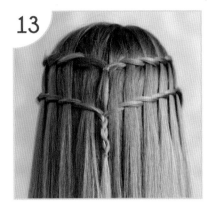

14

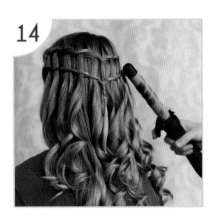

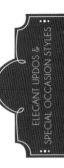

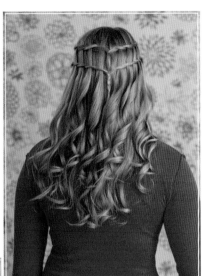

STEP 13 Join the twists together in the middle, and if desired make a micro braid with the ends and secure with an elastic.

STEP 14 For a dressier look and more texture, curl the hair.

QUICK TIP

FOR AN EVEN MORE intricate hairstyle, you can make several more rows of twists below the ones created in this style. Mist entire hairstyle with hair spray.

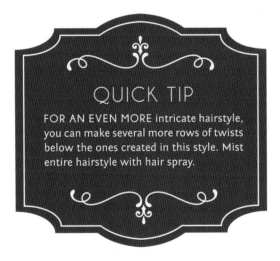

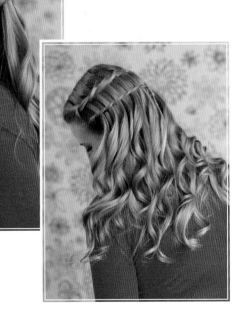

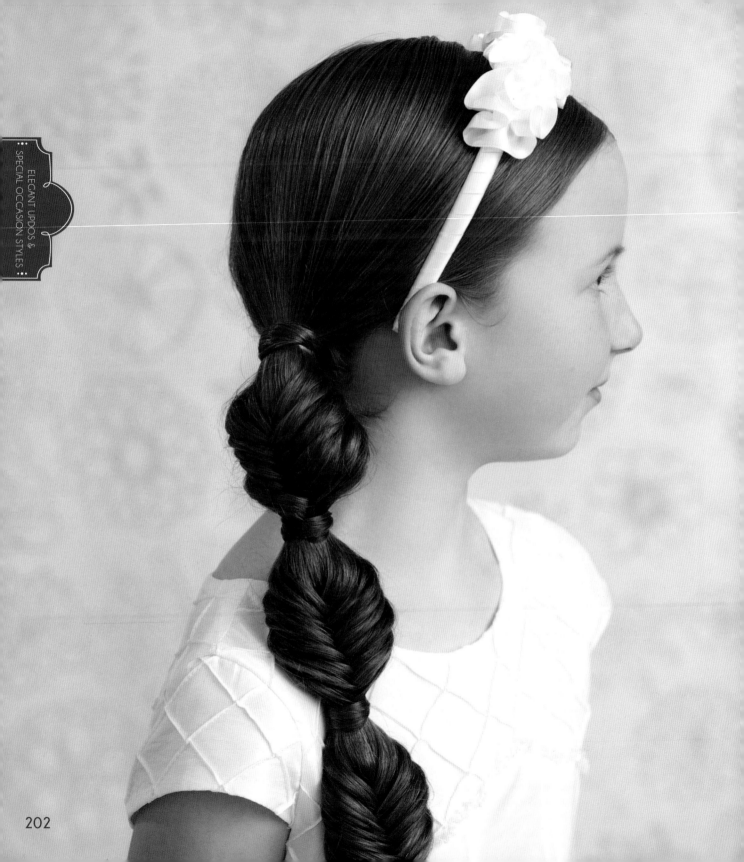

FISHBONE BUBBLES

1

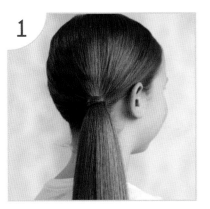

STEP 1 Gather all the hair to the right side of the head and make a low side ponytail behind the right ear. Cover the elastic with hair as shown on page 36.

2

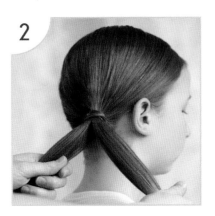

STEP 2 Divide the ponytail into 2 sections.

3

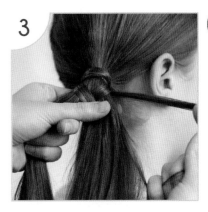

STEP 3 Take small sections of hair from the outer edges and cross them over to the opposite side to create a fishbone braid as shown on page 20.

4

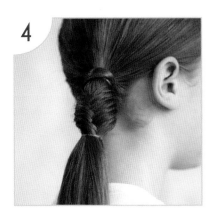

STEP 4 Only plait about 7–8 rotations of the braid and then secure with a clear elastic.

5

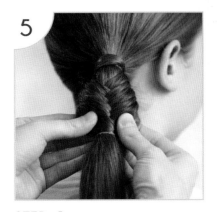

STEP 5 Make this section a bit thicker and wider by gently pancaking the fishbone braid by pulling on the edges of the braid.

6

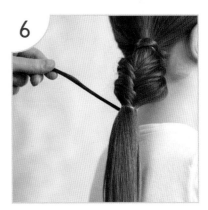

STEP 6 Take a small section of hair from below the elastic and mist with water or hair spray.

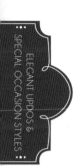

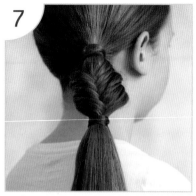

7

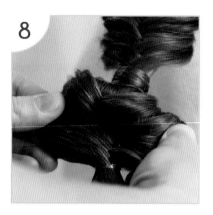

8

STEP 7 Proceed to wrap it around the clear elastic from step 4 and secure the wrapped hair as shown on page 36.

STEP 8 Repeat steps 2–7 two more times (or as many times as desired). Be sure to wrap the very bottom elastic with hair as well.

9A

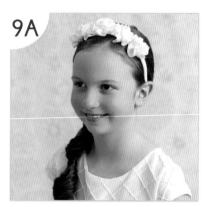

9B

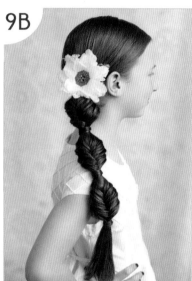

STEPS 9A & 9B Add a pretty headband or other accessory to make the style even fancier. Spray entire hairstyle with hair spray.

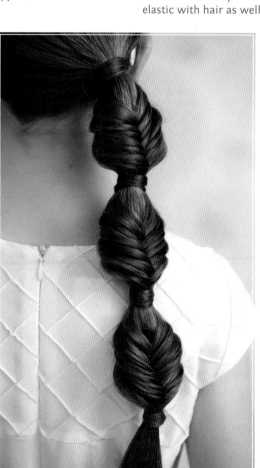

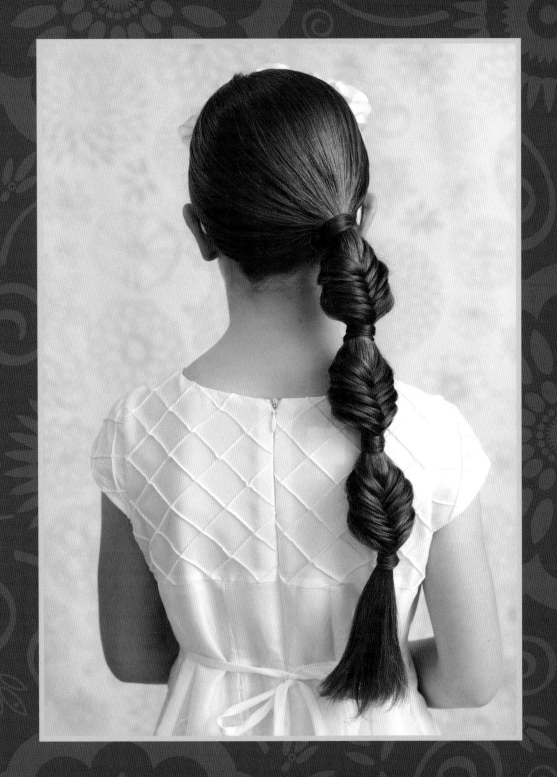

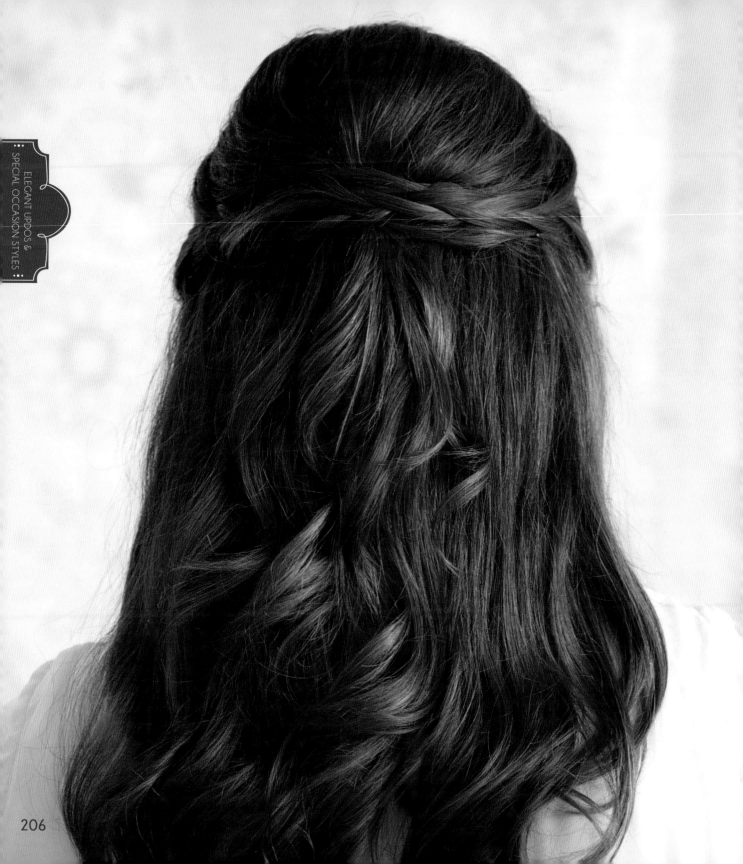

BRAIDED PULLBACK & CURLS

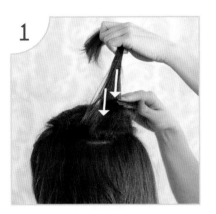

1

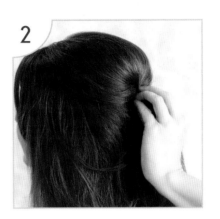

2

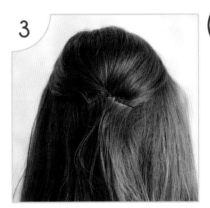

3

STEP 1 From the hairline above the forehead back to the crown, section out small amounts of hair and back comb at the roots to give a bit of volume.

STEP 2 Flip the hair back and smooth the top layer. Gather the hair that was back combed to form a bouffant or "bump" of hair.

STEP 3 Secure this section of hair with a few bobby pins. Overlap the bobby pins to improve the hold.

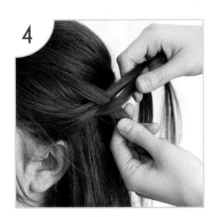

4

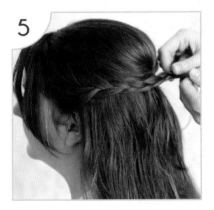

5

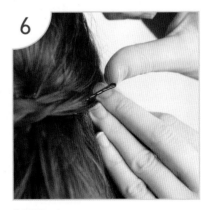

6

STEP 4 Starting on the left side, take the remaining hair by the ear and make a loose regular 3-strand braid (see page 22). Braid until you are a few inches from the end.

STEP 5 Draw the braid to the right across the back of the head, covering the bobby pins.

STEP 6 Secure the braid with a bobby pin on the right side of the bobby pins you just covered up. If the hair you are working with is long enough to extend past the center of the head, leave the tails hanging loose for now.

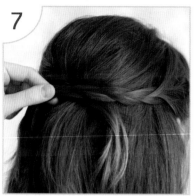

7

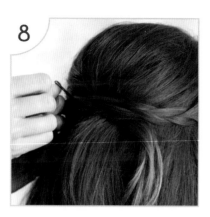

8

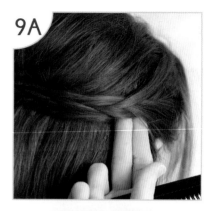

9A

STEP 7 On the right side of the head create another braid with the hair in front of the ear. Draw it back so it lays above the braid from the left side.

STEP 8 Secure the end of the braid on the left side of the bobby pins from Step 3.

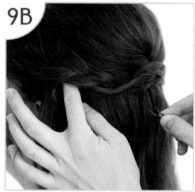

9B

STEPS 9A & 9B With the extra hair from the ends of the braids, gently tuck the tails up under the braids to hide it. If needed, secure with a small bobby pin.

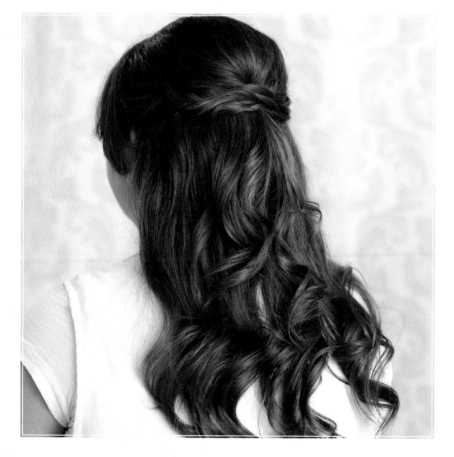

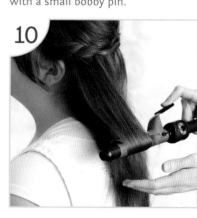

10

STEP 10 Finish the style off by curling the remaining hair in back. Add as little or as much curl as desired and mist with finishing spray.

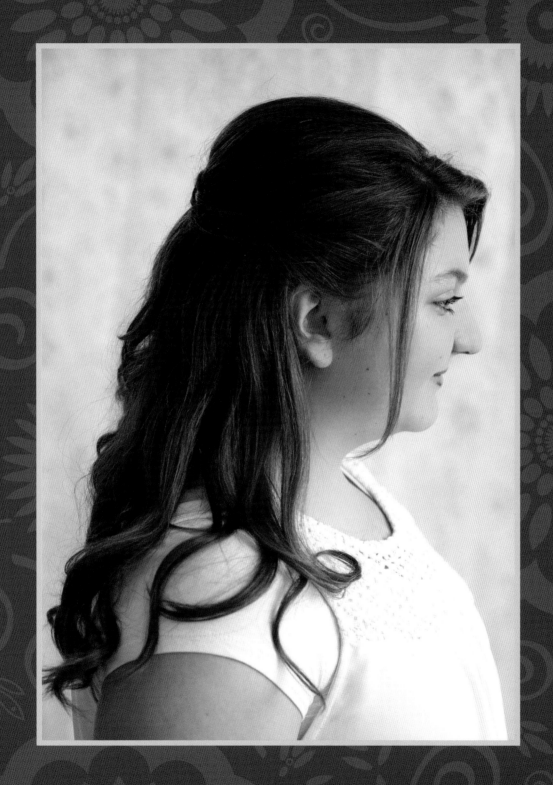

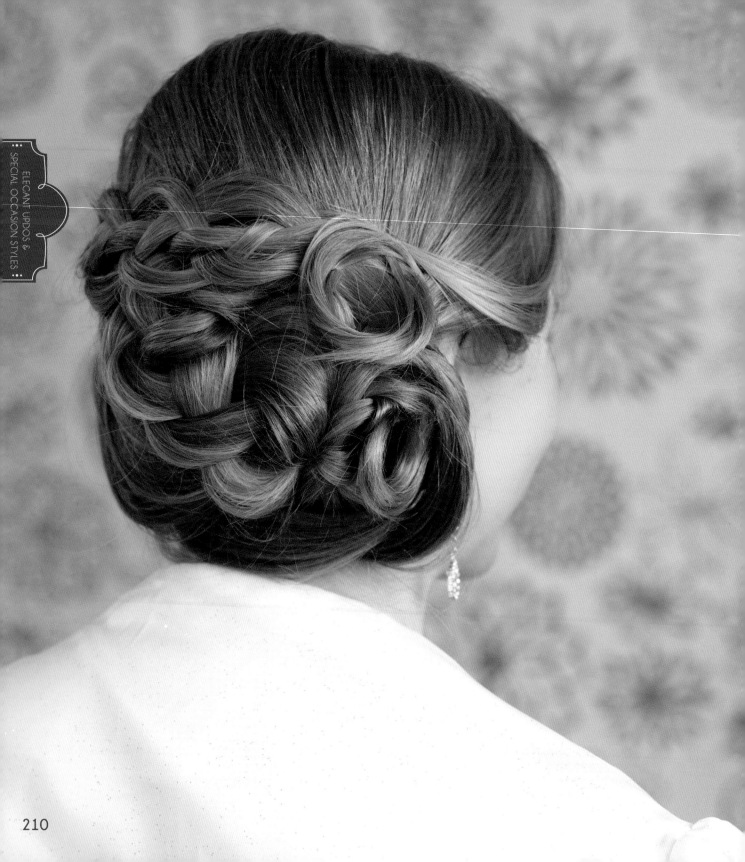

4-STRAND BRAID UPDO

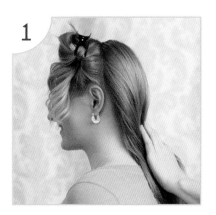

STEP 1 Part the hair on the right side of the head back to the crown. Then from the crown down to the left ear part out that section of hair and temporarily clip out of the way.

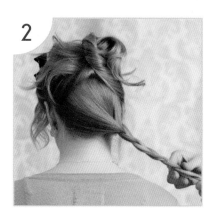

STEP 2 With the remaining hair in back, divide it in half from ear to ear and clip the top section of hair up out of the way. With the rest of the hair that is down, behind the right ear, make a loose 3-strand braid as shown on page 22.

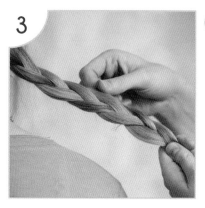

STEP 3 Pull on the edges to slightly pancake the braid and secure the braid at the end with a clear hair elastic.

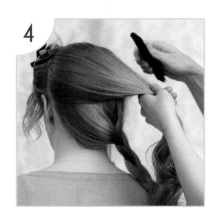

STEP 4 Remove the clip from the section of hair above the braid. Draw the hair to the right side of the head so it is above the braid you just made.

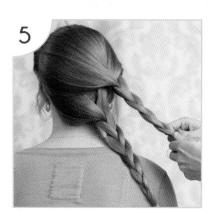

STEP 5 Make another regular 3-strand braid. Pancake it as desired and secure the end of the braid with a clear hair elastic.

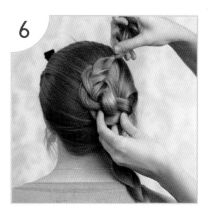

STEP 6 Draw the top braid upward and wrap in a clockwise direction to form a flat bun.

211

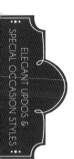

7

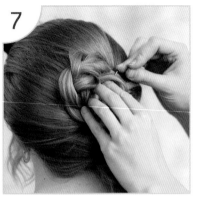

STEP 7 Secure the bun with bobby pins as needed.

8

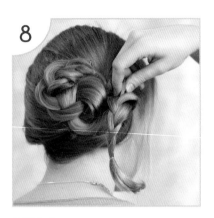

STEP 8 Bring the remaining braid to the right of the bun from Step 6 and wrap in a counterclockwise direction. Lay the braid so the bun resembles a coil or snail shell directly behind the right ear.

9

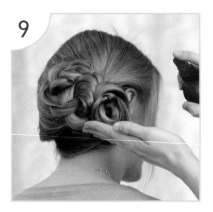

STEP 9 Secure this braid with bobby pins as needed. Try to coil the tail of the braid in the center to give the appearance of a pin curl. Spray with hair spray to keep the tail of the braid in place if needed.

10

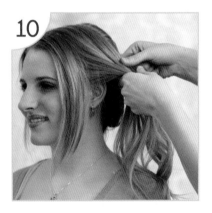

STEP 10 With the remaining hair on the left side, remove the clip and loosely plait a 4-strand braid as shown on page 32. If desired, leave any bangs out of the braid to be drawn back in a later step. Or if preferred, include bangs into this braid.

11

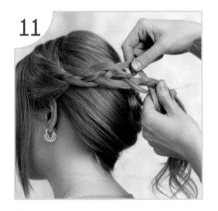

STEP 11 Make the 4-strand braid long enough to reach the right side of the head. Before anchoring the braid, gently pull on the outside sections of the braid to loosen it slightly.

12

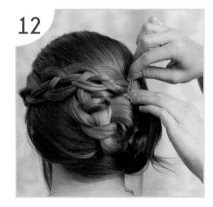

STEP 12 Draw the 4-strand braid to the right side of the head and position it above the bun from step 6. Secure with bobby pins as needed.

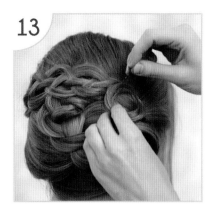

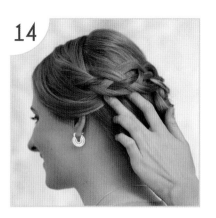

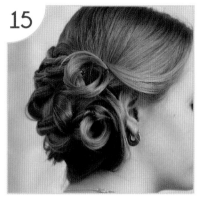

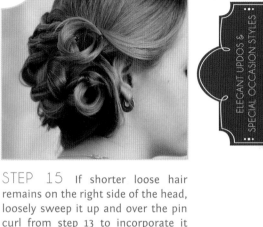

ELEGANT UPDOS &
SPECIAL OCCASION STYLES

STEP 13 With the ends of the hair from the 4-strand braid, carefully wrap them into a pin curl so it forms a circle of hair. It should cover the bobby pin from step 12. Anchor with hair pins as needed.

STEP 14 With the remaining bangs on the left side, draw them back so they cover the top of the left ear and secure with bobby pins under the 4-strand braid.

STEP 15 If shorter loose hair remains on the right side of the head, loosely sweep it up and over the pin curl from step 13 to incorporate it into the style. Secure as needed with hair pins or hair spray. Spray entire style with finishing spray.

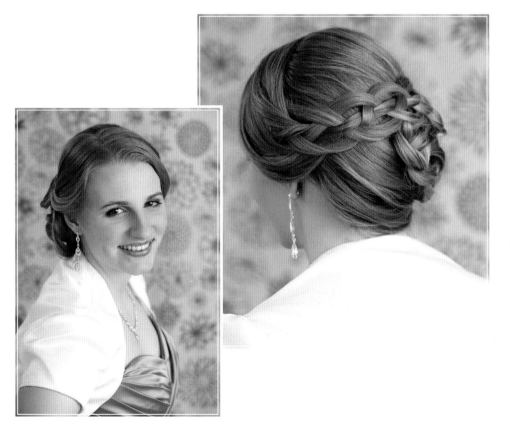

RESOURCES

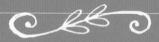

ALL THINGS RIBBON
www.allthingsribbon.com

CURLFORMERS
www.curlformers.com

FAROUK SYSTEMS, INC.—CHI
www.farouk.com

GIMME CLIPS
www.gimmeboutique.com

SALLY BEAUTY SUPPLY
www.sallybeauty.com

INDEX

INDEX

About the
AUTHOR

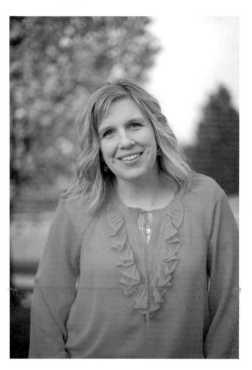

BECKY PORTER is the hands behind the hairstyles. Since starting her blog *Babes In Hairland* (www.babesinhairland.com) in 2008, she has been making the world a prettier place, one head of hair at a time. Besides having a passion for doing hair and teaching hair classes, she loves music, baking, and spending time with her family. She lives in Utah with her three amazing daughters and one patient husband.